NURSING LEADERSHIP:
Theory and Process

NURSING LEADERSHIP:
Theory and Process

Helen Yura, R.N., Ph.D.
ASSISTANT DIRECTOR
DEPARTMENT OF BACCALAUREATE AND HIGHER
DEGREE PROGRAMS
NATIONAL LEAGUE FOR NURSING
NEW YORK, NEW YORK

Dorothy Ozimek, R.N., Ed.D., D.Sci.
DIRECTOR
DEPARTMENT OF BACCALAUREATE AND HIGHER
DEGREE PROGRAMS
NATIONAL LEAGUE FOR NURSING
NEW YORK, NEW YORK

Mary B. Walsh, R.N., M.S.N.
ASSOCIATE PROFESSOR
SCHOOL OF NURSING
THE CATHOLIC UNIVERSITY OF AMERICA
WASHINGTON, D.C.

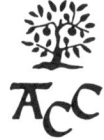

APPLETON-CENTURY-CROFTS/New York
A Publishing Division of Prentice-Hall, Inc.

Library of Congress Cataloging in Publication Data

Yura, Helen.
  Nursing leadership.

  Bibliography: p. 215
  Includes index.
  1. Nursing service administration. 2. Leadership.
I. Ozimek, Dorothy, joint author. II. Walsh,
Mary B., joint author. III. Title. [DNLM: 1.
Leadership. 2. Nursing, Supervisory. 3. Nursing.
WY16 Y95n]
RT89.Y87   610.73   76-10638
ISBN 0-8385-7027-5

Copyright © 1976 by APPLETON-CENTURY-CROFTS
A Publishing Division of Prentice-Hall, Inc.

All rights reserved. This book, or any parts thereof, may not be used or reproduced in any manner without written permission. For information address Appleton-Century-Crofts, 292 Madison Avenue, New York, NY 10017

76 77 78 79 80 / 10 9 8 7 6 5 4 3 2 1

Prentice-Hall International, Inc., London
Prentice-Hall of Australia, Pty. Ltd., Sydney
Prentice-Hall of India Private Limited, New Delhi
Prentice-Hall of Japan, Inc., Tokyo
Prentice-Hall of Southeast Asia (Pte.) Ltd., Singapore

PRINTED IN THE UNITED STATES OF AMERICA

Copyright credits:

Macmillan Publishing Company for permission to use quotations from: Handbook of Leadership, *by Ralph M. Stogdill, 1974 from pages 65, 77, 81, 231, 293 and 344*

Association for Supervision and Curriculum Development for permission to use quotations from: Yearbook 1960 Leadership for Improving Instruction *from page 182*

McGraw-Hill Book Company for permission to use quotations from: Leadership and Organization *by R. Tannenbaum, I. Weschler, and F. Massarik, 1961 from pages 24, 26, 31, and 34*

cover design: Leon Kasmin

DEDICATED
TO

SISTER M. ANTONETTE MARTINKO, MSC

who, as the first nurse leader I knew, continues
to be an inspiration to me

Helen Yura

TO
DR. MILDRED MONTAG

who, as my mentor, exemplified the nursing
leadership process for me

Dorothy Ozimek

TO
WILLIAM AND ELLA BLACKBURN

who, as my parents, provided subtle but sure leadership
which I continue to admire and try to emulate

Mary B. Walsh

Preface

Of major significance to the viability and further development of the profession of nursing is nurturing persons to serve as its leaders. At no time has strong leadership been more significant to the profession of nursing, due to numerous affronts to nursing education and to nursing practice, than during the present.

With this in mind the authors have devoted their energies to exploring the state of nursing leadership and the nursing leadership process: what it is, what it consists of, and its influence on nursing education and practice. The authors are sharing their convictions and observations about nursing leadership based on years of study, observation, and empirical research, as well as personal involvement. Although the content of this book in no way covers the entire subject of nursing leadership, it is hoped that what follows will coordinate what is known and be useful, and, at the same time, stimulate potential and affirmed nurse leaders to test, add to, support, and/or refute the views held in this text.

This book is divided into six chapters. Chapter 1 introduces the topic of leadership in general, with a brief historic review. Surveys of the major contributors to our understanding of leadership and to leadership-related research are included. Factors affecting leadership, such as sex, ability, age, and intelligence are considered; particularly, leadership in nursing is explored. Concepts and theories related to leadership are examined in Chapter 2. These include authority, power, influence, administration, management, and supervision. The third chapter is comprised of the substance of the nursing leadership process. This includes a section on leadership theory, operational definitions of leadership and nursing leadership, the components of the nursing leadership process, a taxonomy of nursing leadership behavior, and the dimensions of nursing leadership behavior as they now exist. The fourth chapter presents a treatise on the educational preparation of the nurse leader. Attention is focused on basic and advanced educational preparation for leadership development. Chapter 5 covers the situational aspects of the nursing leadership process. Situations from nursing education and the nursing service are presented. Chapter 6 outlines the next steps in the development of nursing leadership. A comprehensive bibliography is included for the reader's reference.

The text was written to portray the multidimensional aspects of the nursing leadership process and to suggest a description of what the nursing leadership process is, what it consists of, and how nursing leadership behavior is developed. The most strategic aspects are the identification, development, and nurturing of nurse leaders, and effective utilization of the nursing leadership process. Perhaps any contribution this text may make to understanding the need for the development of nurse leaders, in a deliberate way, will be rewarded by nurses exerting the type and degree of leadership needed to strengthen the profession of nursing and to ensure its future, and ultimately to provide the high quality of nursing care that is needed. The text was written for all nurses interested in the preparation of nurse leaders for the available, required, and unfilled leadership positions in nursing and for the development of those nurses prepared empirically for the leadership positions now filled. Since nurses comprise the largest number of health-care providers in the United States, effective leadership is essential to assure quality health care for persons, families, and communities.

Throughout the text, the term *nurse* refers to a professional nurse whose minimal preparation consists of a baccalaureate degree with an upper division major in nursing. The term *client(s)* is used to mean persons, families, groups of persons, groups of families, or a combination of these, who are well or ill, infirm, injured, disabled, or handicapped, in any setting.

It is recognized that the majority of practicing nurses are women; therefore, the pronoun *she* will be used throughout the text to refer to the nurse. The pronoun *he* is used to refer to the client.

The authors gratefully acknowledge the assistance of many in the preparation of this text. Thanks are due to Dr. Virginia Conley, Dean, School of Nursing, The Catholic University of America, for permission to do the survey reported in the Appendix. Appreciation is extended to the students enrolled in the baccalaureate and masters degree programs in nursing at The Catholic University of America who so generously gave of their time and thoughts and completed the survey forms. The contributions of faculty in NLN accredited baccalaureate and masters degree programs in nursing who unknowingly contributed to this presentation through their submission of self-study reports written to the *Criteria for the Appraisal of Baccalaureate and Higher Degree Programs in Nursing* is acknowledged. Particular acknowledgment is given to Dr. Nan Hechenberger, Associate Professor of Nursing, School of Nursing, University of Maryland, and to Mrs. Elizabeth Ozimek Kaye, Nursing Inservice Education Instructor, New Jersey Neuropsychiatric Institute, Princeton, New Jersey, who so generously shared their views of the nursing leadership process as applied to nursing education and nursing service. Their presentations will be found in Chapter 5. Our appreciation is extended to Richard Miller, who prepared the illustrations.

Special thanks are given to Mary Bersin for her generous assistance and support throughout the preparation of the manuscript and for typing the drafts as well as the completed manuscript.

It has been the authors' privilege to have contributed to the preparation of leaders, as well as to have known and been influenced by great nurse leaders. It is about these persons that this book is written. We hope it will be informative and useful.

Helen Yura
Dorothy Ozimek
Mary B. Walsh

Contents

Preface vii

1 INTRODUCTION 1

2 CONCEPTS AND THEORIES RELATED TO LEADERSHIP 38

3 NURSING LEADERSHIP 82

4 EDUCATIONAL PREPARATION FOR NURSING LEADERSHIP DEVELOPMENT 133

5 SITUATIONAL ASPECTS OF NURSING LEADERSHIP 160

6 NEXT STEPS FOR NURSING LEADERSHIP 194

Appendix 199

Bibliography 215

Index 233

NURSING LEADERSHIP:
Theory and Process

CHAPTER 1
Introduction

Leadership is a fascinating term. It is a positive quality—one to strive for, to seek, to achieve, and to develop. It is a subject discussed by many, a characteristic that seems to be admired by everyone, and easy to recognize in those who possess it. Among siblings, usually one is recognized as the leader. In school playgrounds, leaders emerge from among various play groups; in the classroom, the leader of a group soon becomes apparent. The leader in the classroom however is not necessarily the leader in the playground. Throughout the postsecondary school years, whether in continued education, employment, or any chosen activity, the leader of a group appears. Every social and professional group and all religious and community groups rely on leadership. Political and educational activities are at a standstill unless there is leadership, the essential ingredient of which exists in all activities involving numbers of persons.

Although the English language has included the term *leader* since about the year 1300 and the term leadership since about 1800,[1] shallow inroads have been made in defining the essentials of leadership. Only when these are known can curricula be planned to prepare people to be leaders.

Despite its importance, much is unknown about leadership.

Both an abstract and a real quality, leadership defies simple definition. The multiple definitions available are imprecise and ambiguous. There are numerous synonyms for leadership in the dictionary and others are found in the literature and in actual practice. Each person who uses the term seems to give it individual meaning—few consistent with the others.

Instead of clear phrases that present a verbal picture of leadership, one usually is provided with a litany of characteristics possessed by those who have been recognized as leaders. Descriptions and definitions of leadership are often post facto; one who demonstrates the ability to lead is labeled a leader and his characteristics and traits are itemized in the hope that others will emulate and imitate these traits and they too will become leaders.

There is a paucity of research about leadership. Many professions are experiencing this deficit. For example, one leader in the management area explored the concept of the executive as a leader.[2] As recently as 1967 when his text was published, Peter Drucker reported he had been unable to find a literary discussion or report on how to be an "effective executive."[3] He suggested that effective executives and leaders are scarce and it was his hope that his text would be the first of many writings on the subject. Just as Drucker pursued the subject of leadership among executives, so research and study are necessary to ensure the development of more effective leaders in other areas.

When the literature is explored to find answers to questions about leadership, this term becomes more than fascinating—it becomes intriguing, stimulating, puzzling, confusing, and, most of all, challenging. The more one reads about leadership, the more complex the subject becomes. Its multifaceted nature can be compared to that of a diamond, which has so many sides, so many facets, so many potential approaches from which it can be viewed, that the potential for its study and exploration seems endless. As one facet is explored in depth, the viewer is dazzled by many others on the periphery. So, too, with leadership; as the investigator pursues one dimension, his curiosity is whetted by each of the other multitudes of ideas produced or discovered during the exploration of a single dimension.

Leadership is a popular term in education, and because their audience is susceptible, educators assume a unique responsibility in leadership. However, although they are known for their analytic abilities, research proclivities, and inquiring attitudes, educators have failed to agree on what leadership behaviors are and what the best means are for preparing leaders in the many areas in which they are needed.

Courage is a quality required for leadership. It is particularly important in decision-making and priority setting. While decisions are being made about what is to receive priority in the action arena, posteriorities are also being set. Every posteriority is someone else's top priority.[4] Therefore the leader needs the courage to cope with the perceptions of all. Research studies show that "achievement . . . depends less on research ability than on the courage to go after opportunity." [5]

In Stogdill's superb text on leadership, he has omitted any data about the charismatic leader, stating that although there are many studies about charismatic leaders ". . . comparatively little information is provided that adds to the understanding of leadership." [6] Charisma is probably more intangible than leadership; it is intriguing, although most of us who have experienced charisma have difficulty in "putting our fingers on" just what traits constitute charisma. Certain of our friends exert a charisma that makes us feel better in their presence than in their absence. Some teachers exhibit charisma, felt by some students but not by others; those students, who sense such charisma, can sometimes overcome more obstacles to learning than was ever thought possible. Politicians who possess charisma are very fortunate; their appeal to audiences and constituents is invaluable and gives them a decided edge over opponents who are not as fortunate. Are these persons leaders? Do they possess leadership traits? How can their practices be defined and duplicated? Can charisma be taught? What are the elements of charisma? Published research to date has provided such limited insight into this mercurial trait that it presents an excellent potential for study. If charisma is a trait that improves interpersonal relations, then let it be studied in the laboratory and in the field, to determine what it is and why it works. The fact that no studies are available should not act as a deterrent but rather should stimulate scholars to delve into this unknown area. However, caution must be exercised. Unless charisma is combined with a "down to earth" quality the person responsible for leading will encounter major obstacles. There must be a firm grasp of reality and a clear "understanding of what . . . is going on" in order for charisma to be effective.[7] Some see a contrast between the charismatic (romantic) leader and the more or less commonplace (functional) leader.[8] With the development of technology and a trend toward a more work-oriented society, it is not surprising to note that "in the U.S. . . . the balance between charismatic and pragmatic leadership has usually been weighted toward the latter."[9] President John F. Kennedy probably came close to a blend of both qualities, charisma and pragmatism. It is the exceptional leader who acquires and/or develops either trait with any degree of success. Rare and fortunate indeed is the person who can achieve both.

The essence of American democracy lends itself to the development of leaders and leadership. Americans are known for valuing freedom, opportunity, and democratic decision-making. This American way of life suggests a powerful vitality; it allows for an initiative that is difficult to match.[10] The system of American democracy allows for the development and use of power. The various freedoms enjoyed and exercised by Americans permit them to possess power. Lack of freedom removes such power from the individual and it then originates in another person who has control over that individual depriving him of his freedom.[11]

Giving a person power imposes certain obligations; as a superior, he is responsible for the work of others; also, he has power over their careers.[12] The equivalent duty of the one holding such power is to observe justice and respect the individuality of each follower in the group.

History records the feats of persons labeled as leaders. Scrutiny of such persons reveals some traits held in common; it also reveals some very disparate characteristics. Napoleon and Hitler were recognized as leaders, especially valuable in time of war. Both were small in stature, a physical characteristic that most research studies state is inconsistent with leadership. A review of American history reveals that in the majority of U.S. Presidential elections, the taller of the two major party candidates won the election. Is it possible that the physical characteristic of tall stature is pertinent to the United States only? Columbus was a leader—a daring, adventurous person who faced unknown dangers as he sailed from Spain to discover the "New World." Perhaps his courage is the significant synonym for leadership. Churchill was not considered very successful until he found his niche during World War II. His leadership provided England with a "lamp of hope" during very dark days. Certainly his age was not a deterrent to his effective leadership.

Although Warren Harding's success as President can be debated, he was described as "preternaturally erect, . . . looked . . . a leader of men." [13] In addition to his physical attributes, he was an articulate speaker who could successfully woo audiences. President Kennedy, too, was tall and had a regal bearing; he was articulate, possessed a certain charisma, and had an appropriate sense of humor. James Cardinal Gibbons was a paradox among leaders. "His mind was unoriginal . . . he sponsored no major projects on his own initiative . . . was a mediocre orator . . . a colorless writer"; was of "medium height, exceptionally thin," yet he was an "extraordinary man and the greatest figure the church has produced in America." [14] His major strength was diplomacy.

Despite efforts to include leadership in various curricula, a major variable is the background of each person who hopes, or expects, to become a leader. Early experiences with figures in authority influence the person who is moving into a leadership role. The exact amount of influence is difficult to measure or predict, but there is evidence that such influence exists. How one can be expected to relate to persons in leader–follower situations depends upon his or her childhood experiences with authority figures, such as parents, teachers, ministers, and others.[15]

The influence of cultural groups is inescapable, also. Certain ethnic groups deal with authority in their own specific ways. For example, a German family may view the father role quite differently from a British family. Germans refer to Germany as the "Fatherland"; the British refer to Britain as the "Motherland," the Russian calls his country the "Homeland," and the American generally refers to the United States as "Our land." Each of these persons approaches leadership situations influenced not only by his country of origin but also by his family and social experiences during his developing years.

The complex facets of leadership have many dimensions. Systematic studies are needed to clarify specific influences. The terms leader and leadership need to be defined precisely. The various fields of functioning and the various professions should assume responsibility for specifying leadership behaviors and for identifying the route to assist persons in acquiring desirable leadership traits. There are a number of challenging variables operating in the study of leadership, namely, physical characteristics, personal traits, such as charisma, articulate speaking ability, sense of humor, courage, family and life experiences, and family heritage.

Finally, the eye of the beholder adds a further dimension that will also be difficult to evaluate. Each person perceives events according to his own orientation and according to the view he holds of the situation or event. President Truman observed that two people seldom perceive the same event in exactly the same way. He expressed his admiration for the stories in the Bible, especially the Gospels. He noted the ". . . way those fellas saw the same things in a different manner . . . and they were all telling the truth . . . no two people ever see the same thing in quite the same way, and when they tell it the way they saw it, they aren't necessarily lying if it's different." [16]

LEADERSHIP IN NURSING

Like many other professions, nursing "bemoans its lack of leadership." [17] The thirty-year period since World War II has been a time of accelerated change in all areas of nursing. Nursing leadership has not been excluded nor exempt from these changes.

Immediately following World War II, the levels and numbers of auxiliary personnel in nursing began to increase greatly. As a result activities previously considered the sole responsibility of the professional nurse were performed by auxiliary personnel. Therefore, it became necessary to organize these personnel into groups so that assigned tasks could be performed more efficiently; the professional nurse, as the person who had the most preparation for nursing, became the leader of the groups. As the nurses were assigned more responsibility for the organization and management of activities necessary for patient care, they became more aware of their need for added preparation in the area of leadership.

During the 1950s, even greater emphasis was placed on preparing professional nurses for positions variously called supervisor, administrator, or manager.[18] Heretofore, most of the leadership behaviors employed by professional nurses were learned "on the job," through the apprentice system, and by trial and error. Despite the inadequacies inherent in this type of preparation, many fine managers evolved. However, many nurses were lost to the profession because of their frustration in having responsibilities thrust upon them that they had not been prepared to meet through education or experience.

Not long after educational programs for administrators got underway, another trend in nursing appeared. Educational programs began to change from a functional to a clinical goal. The shift in direction was not sudden; it was a sure and gradual change that eventually occurred in all accredited educational programs. The intention was not to negate or ignore the need for leadership ability, but to add to the responsibilities of the professional nurse. Not only was it neccesary for the nurse to occupy a leader role, but in order to lead other personnel involved in the care of clients, she also had to be proficient and knowledgeable in clinical nursing, teaching techniques, and curriculum content.

Leadership skills needed by the nurse expanded beyond those required to direct only her own activities to the multifaceted responsibilities of directing increasing numbers of health-oriented personnel with ever widening levels of preparation.

A change was also taking place in the client population. Historically, clients were a submissive group of persons who followed the directions of professional and ancillary nursing personnel, without doubt or question. Today, increased knowledge about health is available to the lay public. As this knowledge has accumulated, health care consumers have become responsible for an increased amount of their own care. This has changed the type of client with whom the nurse functions; it has brought a new challenge to nursing and has given a different dimension to health care than was present in the past. The nurse continues to function as the leader of health care practices for clients, but she is not experiencing blind followership; rather she has followers who are knowledgeable, alert, and questioning—who know they have legal rights—and who are not reluctant to exercise these rights. The pace of change today continues to accelerate. Changes are occurring so rapidly that it is difficult to precisely ascribe one or even a few causes for any one change. In this text we will identify some of the major changes that have had an impact on nursing leadership, but no attempt will be made to align them with all causes for change.

The setting in which the client is located is of major importance to the nurse. Hospitals are focusing more directly on care of the acutely ill and the role of this client is less powerful than that of clients outside the hospital walls. Because the client is acutely ill, the nurse acts as leader of the health group by performing as a client advocate. In the role of leader she is performing acts for the client which, because of his illness, he is unable to do for himself. This requires astute perception of the client's needs as well as the ability to accurately communicate these needs to other persons involved in his care.

On the other hand, many settings exist outside the hospital where the role of the client is more autonomous and more independent than in the hospital setting. These may include a clinic, the client's home, a physician's office, a community health fair, or a variety of settings. In such settings, the nurse occupies the role of leader, using the same skills of leadership as in the hospital setting, but adapting these skills to the language, interests, and needs of the client, according to variables in environment.

As man's life span continues to increase, the nurse is confronted with the need to adapt leadership behaviors to a growing number of older persons. The physical and behavioral changes that occur with aging are well known. Changes in vision, hearing, mobility, circulation, digestion, elimination, and in the nervous system create a different focus and pace for the client. Mood swings and emotional responses present patterns with which the client's family is trying to cope. The nurse faces the challenge of helping the client to cope with his own needs, helping the family to understand what is happening and why, and how best to adapt and adjust to evidences of health deviations. Difficult decisions, laden with emotional impact and psychologic trauma are often more stressful than responsibility for physical care. Families are faced with decisions about nursing home versus their own home for a disabled or an older family member. Providing support and empathy as they labor through such a difficult process requires more conscious leadership than is often required in administering physical care. Through careful and deliberate leadership, the nurse can be helpful to the client and family. She can also set the important standards of quality care by seizing this opportunity to demonstrate positive and constructive leadership ability.

It is primarily in hospital settings and health care agencies that the various types of leadership are discussed. Although some modification of these kinds of leadership is employed in any setting, directive or autocratic types are usually contrasted with creative or democratic types. Seldom is either type seen to the total exclusion of the other, but one usually predominates. Directive leadership is less popular because there is little or no input from group members; all decision making, goal setting, planning, and evaluation are done by the leader.[19] This style of leading stifles motivation and creativity, limits job satisfaction or a sense of achievement, and prohibits any evaluation among group members. Democratic leadership poses responsibilities for the leader as well as group members. It is usually a longer process, requiring more time to realize results, but utilizes resources of the group as a whole for the benefit of the client and is more productive and satisfying to a group of nurses. The nurse uses different skills when functioning as a democratic group leader compared to functioning as an autocrat. Patience and tolerance of the democratic process are virtues that must be encouraged and developed by the nurse leader.

In an effort to arrive at a plan in which all levels of personnel could be used the concept called "team nursing" has been tried for a number of years. Essentially, this is a plan of organization in which the professional nurse is responsible for the care of a selected number of clients. A specified number of other nurses and/or nursing personnel are assigned to assist with such care. Central to the team concept was the idea that the professional nurse was the person held responsible for client care; assignments of care and activities were made by the professional nurse; conferences were held to ensure communication among team members about the care of clients. The chief benefit derived from the team method of assignment was the increased amount of supervision available to the nonprofessional personnel under such a system.

Within the team method of nursing, assignments were made according to either functional or case methods. These methods of assignments were often used outside, or instead, of team nursing. The team leader or the professional nurse "in charge" could sometimes choose the method of assignment, but most frequently, a directive from the nursing office indicated the method. In such instances, the creativity and motivation of the team leaders were ignored or not considered important.

One innovation that occurred soon after team nursing was initiated was unit managers or ward managers. This step was an effort to employ a person (nonnurse) to perform the technical details and paper work necessary for the functioning of a hospital unit so that nursing personnel could devote full time and energy to direct client care activities. In some situations, the unit manager and team nursing systems were efficient and effective. In other situations, these systems created only chaos and discontent among both staff and client groups.

As the needs of clients continue to change and grow in complexity, and as nursing continues to try various methods and maneuvers to cope with client needs, the challenge to provide keen leadership grows. With primary nursing appearing in the professional arena, the advent of increasing specialization, the growing popularity of "nurse practitioners," and so much attention to the expanding functions or responsibilities of the nurse, it seems essential that in each setting or area where there are clients, there should be a nurse leader to guide and direct the group toward specific and defined goals. With increasing frequency, the terms *nurse leader* and *nursing leadership* are being heard. Many persons who use these terms are sure of their meaning; others are not as sure, but the terms sound good and are sophisticated. They seem to say something that requires and demands respect.

Efforts in nursing education over the past few years have been directed toward defining conceptual frameworks and theoretical foundations on which many of nursing's heretofore instinctive practices can be placed. Leadership is a concept that permeates all of professional nursing. It is a concept that can be described by rather specific behaviors. Identifying desirable leadership behaviors enables the teacher to plan the nursing curriculum in such a way that concepts, theories, and behaviors of leadership are essential parts of the curriculum. The intended goal of professional nurses prepared as educated leaders of nursing will then be realized.

NURSING LEADERSHIP RESEARCH

Among the many activities in which nurses are involved, perhaps the most formidable is research. Whether it is the nature of the research, or limited interest in this field for a variety of reasons, some nurses do not find it attractive. There is much potential for research in nursing, however. While reflecting on the many fertile research fields, the rather obvious route for involving nurses in such studies is to have leaders in nursing point the way. A number of persons are identified or recognized as leaders in nursing, but when the area of leadership in nursing is explored, the paucity of published studies in this subject area becomes immediately apparent.

Leadership is a current concern. Dorothy Kelly suggests that it "seems to be building toward a major issue in nursing." [20] The lack of published data about nursing leadership substantiates Kelly's view. Any discerning observer can view the need for leadership in a patient or client setting, whether a hospital or community agency. In some instances, the need for leadership is being adequately filled, yet in other instances, sound and efficient leadership is sorely needed.

As the astute observer becomes more involved in exploring

nursing leadership, the cry, "we need some leadership" becomes louder. Perhaps Kelly is correct in precisely diagnosing the problem as one that is in need of good followers as well as good leaders.[21] Both elements, leader and follower, are necessary in any situation: Unless both exist, leadership cannot develop or occur. Should the plea in professional nursing be, "We need some followers as well as leaders?" In the continual struggle to teach others to lead, nurses have been no more successful than other groups in following the theory of the leadership traitists. Proponents of this theory feel that if one describes or defines the traits of a person who is recognized as a leader, others will imitate and emulate these enunciated traits, and presto, a new leader emerges.[22] As the explosion of knowledge continues to accelerate, as the numbers of persons who populate the world increases, and as the United States citizenry, in particular, becomes more conscious of its health needs, the need for more efficient nursing leadership becomes obvious.

The limited amount of research in nursing leadership poses a handicap; yet it is not an insurmountable one. The elements of research are now being taught in qualitative nursing educational programs; this preparation is fortifying the profession with the means of resolving a major dilemma, that of defining the elements of nursing leadership so that nurses can be taught to be effective leaders.

Although several approaches to research in nursing leadership are possible, three potential areas for study are:

1. Nursing leadership from the client's perspective;
2. Nursing leadership from the perspective of the practicing nurse;
3. Nursing leadership from the perspective of the nursing student.

A review of the recent literature reveals that some authors have reported their interest and efforts in studies related to nursing leadership.

The student of nursing is a worthy candidate for an area of inquiry. Meleis and Farrell reported a study in which the population consisted of 188 students in 6 schools in the San Francisco area; they were enrolled in three programs—the baccalaureate, the associate degree, and the diploma.[23] The students were tested in several areas, one of which was leadership. Fleischmann's Leadership Opinion

Questionnaire was used to test the area of leadership and the students' opinions were compared.[24] The investigators concluded that despite the type of program in which the students were enrolled, all scored essentially alike in the "consideration" * aspect of leadership. When the "structure" † and "autonomy" factors of leadership were compared, however, baccalaureate students rated higher in these areas than students enrolled in the other two types of programs.

When published reports of studies directed to the subject of nursing leadership are reviewed, a number of variables are perceived that can influence leadership behaviors. Practicing nurses are able to identify variables and factors crucial to the practice of leadership, specifically nursing leadership.

One such variable was identified and investigated by Greenfield and Kassum.[25] The style of leadership employed by 82 female employees was studied to identify the leadership style used and to determine which style contributed most effectively to the purposes of the organization. The styles identified were:

1. Consideration (concern for people)
2. Initiating structure (concern for production)

It was concluded that effective supervision requires a high level of both styles. Unless there is concern for the individual who is the employee, the task is not likely to be accomplished. The concern for production or task orientation takes on meaning as important as concern for the employee, and vice versa.

Kelly studied a group of 545 registered nurses employed in a hospital setting.[26] The investigation was intended to predict the leadership potential of the population as a basis for promotion. Forty-two of those tested were actually promoted and the traits common to this group were identified. Three decisive traits in the promoted group were: capacity for status, femininity, and a relaxed manner. The latter trait (a relaxed manner) was used synonymously with poise.

---

* "Consideration" reflects the extent to which a person is likely to have job relationships with his subordinates characterized by mutual trust, respect for their ideas, consideration of their feelings, and a certain warmth between them.

† "Structure" is the extent to which a person is apt to define and structure his own role and those of his subordinates toward goal attainment.

Another variable that has intrigued nurse researchers is a nurse's selection of clinical areas in which to practice. For example, the study by Lois Lukens compared the personality patterns of nurses who chose psychiatric nursing as a field of practice compared to those who chose medical–surgical nursing.[27] A number of differences in patterns were identified and certain needs for knowledge were specified for each of the populations in the study.

Gilbert studied a group of medical–surgical and psychiatric nursing graduate students to determine their leadership potential.[28] Tools for the study were the California Psychological Inventory and the Managerial Key for the California Psychological Inventory. Gilbert found that both groups of nurses scored high on the leadership potential test.

A fascinating area for some research in nursing is that related to motivation and the nurse. Maslow suggests that the level of a person's complaints can suggest the motivational level of that person.[29] For example, if nurses are working in a situation such as a flood disaster, the basic needs of the afflicted as well as those of the workers are of primary concern. Complaints about problems that interfere with meeting the very elementary physiologic needs will be of a "low grumble" character. In another nursing situation (in a modern hospital unit), these basic needs are provided for and the low level grumble is not heard. Rather, power struggles may be going on; dignity and self-respect may be violated; prestige may be threatened; grumbles are on a high level. These are labeled "high grumbles." Further along the hierarchy, some nurses may be concerned with justice; for example, efforts are not being rewarded, sacrifices not being recognized. These complaints suggest that other needs, more basic ones, are being satisfied, and the concerns are matters on a much higher scale than basic needs.[30] Perhaps a study to determine the level at which most nurses grumble would suggest just how healthy the nursing profession is at present, at least from the standpoint of levels of grumbles. Perhaps a correlation between leadership and grumbling could be identified.

Motivation theory suggests that complaints among persons will never cease; instead they will move among levels, depending on specific situations and variables in the situation.[31] So, too, frustration levels can be expected, but not operating at identical levels all the time. Rather, basic needs will determine levels of motivation and frustration according to the perception of a work situation and role in that situation.

It has been suggested that various points in behavioral science have been emphasized in the past four decades.[32] In the 1940s human relations were emphasized; in the 1950s it was participative management; T-groups were the focus in the 1960s; the 1970s are now stressing job enrichment.[32] Pursuing fads of the current decade, determining personality variables that enhance or deter leadership, looking at the personality of the nurse leader, determining whether the nursing leader is person or organization oriented, or whether and how the role of student, teacher, or employee affects one's leadership ability, or how the client perceives the nurse, or vice versa, are among the many potential areas for study. Some inroads have been made in the study of nursing leadership but there are still many more to be done.

INFLUENTIAL FACTORS IN LEADERSHIP

The dilemma in the field of nursing is a result of a narrow, constricted view of leadership and leaders in nursing situations, coupled with a lack of adequately prepared and a sufficient number of leaders. A basic reason for the absence of nurse leaders is the failure to prepare or permit educationally prepared professional nurses to function as leaders. Most employers of nurses persist in regarding them and the practice of nursing as based upon task-oriented skills. The procedures to be performed by nurses are dictated by bureaucratic forces with a vision of concern limited to the needs of the institution rather than the health and nursing care needs of clients, families, and communities.

Leadership is inherent in the professional practice of nursing where the primary goal is care of clients and families. The leaders and leadership in nursing, as presently envisioned, are restricted almost exclusively to hierarchic positions on an organizational chart in institutions that provide nursing services and nursing education.

Nursing service and education are the two major situational environments of nursing. Dimensions of the leadership process are the functions of the professional role of nursing and they are utilized in any and all social settings as well as in any and all fields of nursing. The nurse assumes the lead in defining and planning nursing in any situation regardless of bureaucratic and organizational structure.

The position of the nurse in the health care delivery system is one of the most difficult in society. The nurse is accountable to four distinct and interrelated publics that make a variety of contradictory demands upon her. A professional nurse is responsible first and, most importantly, to her clients, then to her employing institution, to her colleagues and subordinates, and lastly to other members of the health care team. In the present structure for the delivery of health services, the nurse is expected to be accountable in this order of priority; first, to the administrative staff of her employer; then to the physician and other nurses; lastly to the most important member of the quadrangle, the clients in her care. Nursing has been guilty of promoting conformists and followers who bend to fit the existing system even though they know and were taught to consider the client's interests as paramount. The discipline of nursing suffers from a dearth of prepared leaders who are independent, innovative, and creative, and who are motivated to change the health care delivery system so that persons, families, and communities are primary.

Nursing leaders are needed as practitioners, educators, consultants, administrators, researchers, theorists, and clinical specialists. Intangible though leadership may be, we strongly believe that our colleges and universities can design curriculums to develop needed leaders in nursing. Nursing requires leaders who will see that the health care needs of the people come first.

According to the most up-to-date research and as mentioned earlier, no one trait or characteristic of behavior is indicative of leadership. Effectiveness and success in leadership is seen as an interrelationship of the personality traits, characteristics, and behaviors of the leader, the follower, and the situational aspects that are the environment where leadership is effected. Stogdill states that theorists no longer explain leadership solely in terms of the individual or group. Rather, it is believed that characteristics of the individual and demands of the situation interact in such a manner as to permit one or perhaps a few individuals to rise to the leadership status.[33] In the distant past and even to the beginning of this century, leaders were thought to be superior individuals who, as a result of inheritance or social advantages, had qualities and abilities different than those of others. Although much of the literature related to the theory and practice of leadership makes it rather explicit that leadership is situationally centered, the fact remains leaders and leadership are contingent upon more than particular factors of a given situation. To demonstrate what leadership means and how it operates, and to learn how to be a leader, it is important to understand all influencing factors related to leadership. In order to prepare and continue to develop nurse leaders, the factors that appear to influence leadership and the special competencies that leaders should possess must be identified.

The 1960 Yearbook of the Association for Supervision and Curriculum Development was devoted to a study of leadership for improving instruction. In the preparation of the yearbook, 500 research studies were reviewed and provided basic information related to leadership in general. The most fundamental information related to leadership was stated to be the following:

1. Leadership is a product of the interaction that takes place among individuals in a group and not of the status or position of these individuals. Status assignments may enhance or reduce the effectiveness of leader behavior.
2. All group members have leadership potential and exhibit leadership behavior to some degree. Leadership potential is not centered in one or two persons in a group.
3. Behaviors that help a person to be a leader in one situation may not work equally well in others. Because a person exhibits leader behaviors in one group does not guarantee that he can or will do so in others. Leadership shifts from situation to situation.
4. The effectiveness of leader behavior is measured in terms of mutuality of goals, productivity in the achievement of these goals and the maintenance of group solidarity.[34]

With this statement of basic information, let us briefly review traits and characteristics. Traits and characteristics are defined as distinguishing features. The features of a leader will be subdivided into physical, social, intellectual, and personality traits and characteristics. Many studies have been conducted to measure the physical characteristics of successful leaders to discover if leaders have physical distinctions. The major studies were concerned with age, height, weight, activity, and appearance. Age was not found to correlate with leadership. Findings relative to age were that creative persons exhibit the ability to lead at an early age, but our society waits for leaders to acquire the administrative know-how that comes with experience. Few persons are granted leader status in our culture until they reach middle age. In a reply to those who equate age and wisdom, an astute observer once suggested that if one is not particularly wise during his growing and maturing years, he is not apt to be wise in his older years. So too with leadership ability—it does not happen miraculously as one becomes mature, but needs to be developed over the course of a lifetime.

An interesting fact regarding age and leaders that is germane to the profession of nursing (a field predominantly made up of women) is that girl leaders tend to be younger than boy leaders when compared to nonleaders of both sexes. A recent Tel-News release from the New Jersey Bell Telephone Company contained this note that indicates little change in the past 100 years:

> Cornelia Hancock of Hancocks Bridge wasn't daunted when she was turned down as a nurse during the Civil War because of her "youth and rosey cheeks." It was considered "indecorous for angels of mercy to appear otherwise than gray haired and spectacled" but the stubborn 23-year-old arrived at the Gettysburg battlefield in 1863 to care for the wounded anyway. And within a year she'd received such wide acclaim for bravery and devotion to the Union troops that the Secretary of War honored her with a pass to visit anywhere in the lines of the Union Army.[35]

Above average height and weight within a peer group appear to be an advantage. However, according to Stogdill, results of recent research suggest that the leader tends to be endowed with an abundant reserve of energy, stamina, and ability to maintain a high rate of physical activity. Even when handicapped by physical disability or poor health, the successful leader tends to exhibit a high rate of energy output.[36] The evidence presented in the literature reviewed suggested a possible relationship between appearance and leadership, yet recent studies show comparatively little concern with the physical characteristics and appearance of leaders.

A leader is a social being who is an active participant in a great variety of activities, interacts easily, cooperates, can induce cooperativeness, and fosters loyalty and group cohesiveness. The leader is characterized by effective interpersonal skills that include tactfulness. Stogdill compared all surveys of leadership characteristics from 1948 through 1970 and drew the following conclusions related to social factors:

> (1) high socioeconomic status is an advantage in attaining leadership status; (2) leaders who rise to high level positions in industry tend to come from lower socioeconomic strata of society at present than they did a half century ago, and (3) they tend to be better educated than formerly.[37]

We would be remiss if information related to gender was excluded from a consideration of social factors since the feminist movement is a prominent social force at present. Even though gender does not affect one's ability to lead or nurse, information related to the present place of women as leaders must be reviewed. Women populate the United States in greater numbers than men and are reported to possess most of the nation's wealth. Women are still number two (but trying harder to assert themselves) in providing direction for the country in social, health, economic, and political matters. *Time* magazine reported the following related to the place of women. In politics, 1974 was the "year of the woman." [38] Connecticut elected a woman as Governor. Gains were made by women in the United States Congress with an increase of a few seats in the House of Representatives. More women tried for state legislative offices. There were 1200 women candidates on state ballots and more than one-half were elected. A few were nurses. What are the professions that are purported to produce the country's leaders? How are women faring? The American Bar Association stated that women make up 7 percent of the 400,000 lawyers practicing in the United States. This represents an increase from 2.8 percent in 1972.[39] It was also reported that women are entering medicine in greater numbers than in most other professions. It was reported that in the fall of 1974 twenty-five percent of the nation's incoming medical students were women, up from 13 percent in 1972.[39]

Time stated that a more mature feminism has come to focus on the drive for equality on the job, in the home, and in the nation's political life.[39] There were impressive gains to indicate that feminism is far from a fad as was once believed; it is a strong and enduring social force. The progress of women is and will continue to be hampered by tokenism, chauvinism, and women's reluctance to abandon submissive and dependent roles. The nurse who would be a leader must also abandon the submissive dependent role. Unless women stop bending to fit the system and give up conformity, the real "year of the woman" and an abundance of nurse leaders is far off. The women's movement and nurses and nurse leadership are inextricably interwoven. At the 1975 National Student Nurse Association Convention in April, a resolution was passed by the potential future leaders of nursing regarding the rights and responsibilities of women in nursing. The final resolution follows:

> Resolved that women assert equality by accepting full challenges and responsibilities they share with men as part of the decision making mainstream of American political, economic and social life. National Student Nurse Association will discourage and openly fight any manifestations of discrimination and will through publication, encouragement and other action raise the consciousness of all student nurses so that they may most effectively create a new image of women.[40]

No research was reviewed that considered gender in relation to leadership. However, research does suggest that girls are reared in a way that severely constricts their motivational development in realizing their full intellectual competence and leadership abilities. Notions of femininity have greatly hindered women's capacity to be assertive, active, and independent. The question remains: Why have women made virtually no progress in assuming positions of leadership and authority? A partial answer has to do with discriminative policies in employment. Nurses have risen to positions of leadership and authority within the field of nursing, but few have achieved such positions outside the field of nursing, in the total health care field, or in the field of education. Children learn that it is healthy and normal for men and women to function in hierarchical pairs with men as the leaders and initiators and women as followers and helpers. A case in point is the present movement to utilize professional nurses (mainly women) as physician extenders. Physicians are mostly men; they maintain the lead and initiate health and nursing care; the nurse still follows and helps the physician.

A woman who aspires to assume leadership and interact in a forceful, intelligent, assertive, and independent manner pays a price. In adolescence she is told she is a "tomboy"; as an adult she will hear that she is domineering, castrating, and competitive; forever she will be labeled "unladylike." The public is still unable to recognize that a person's place in society should be determined by talent, knowledge, capacity, and inclination rather than by simplistic gender stereotypes.

History resounds with the names of women as leaders from the biblical Deborah who led the Israelites to victory, Egypt's Nefertiti, France's Joan of Arc, and England's Elizabeth I down to modern women. The 1970s alone have produced no fewer than four female heads of state—Israel's Golda Meir, India's Indira Gandhi, Sri Lanka's Sirimavo Bandaranacke, and Argentina's Isabelita Peron. They are clearly the exceptions, however. Women have made amazing progress, but they are hardly present in any numbers as great world leaders. The revolution in the real status of women is only in its infancy. Although discrimination by men has a great deal to do with the small number of women leaders, women's self-concepts are significant obstacles. Leadership in all areas of life will come for women when society has erased sex stereotypes. There are myths about the different and inferior ways in which females perform that relate to the picture of the woman in the home that most men hold in their minds and carry to other environments. Men, who are the gatekeepers to most of the positions of power and authority, think of women in their roles of mother and wife, which are separate and distinct. Wife and mother are functional roles that require an abundance of leadership ability for self-fulfillment, child and husband development, and family stability.

What are the most patent myths about women? Women are too emotional; they will not work for other women; they are too passive to be leaders or, conversely, they become too aggressive and "unfeminine" in positions of power; they have high absenteeism and turnover rates on the job; they are best suited to certain kinds of work. The desire of women to reach their full potentials in no way means that they should assume the dominant role over men. The roles of people—men and women—should be as relative equals in all fields of endeavor—the labor market, the professions, and politics. In the leadership role, a leader (man or woman) leads and draws upon the fullest capabilities of followers, but never assumes the role of master or exhibits mastery over others. As in a democracy, leadership requires collaboration between leaders and those led, regardless of the sex of the leader or follower.

Many factors contribute to the emergence of a leader. Among the factors are intelligence and ability. Stogdill found that leaders are characterized by superior judgment, decisiveness, knowledge, and fluency of speech.[41] It is interesting to note that the general trend of the findings show that superior intelligence is a detriment rather than an absolute requirement for leadership.[41] Authorities on leadership traits find that people seem to desire to be led by the average person who is not too far detached from the group. The leader's contributions and communications must be understood by followers. Factors in the intellectual realm associated with leadership are verbal facility, judgment, knowledge, insight, and scholarship. Leaders made better than average scholastic grades and were more intelligent on the average than nonleaders.

Personality traits have been found to differentiate leaders from followers; however, tests designed to measure different aspects of personality for the selection of leaders have not proved predictive or useful, according to Stogdill.[42] Personality characteristics that appeared to distinguish leaders were alertness, originality, personal integrity, and confidence. The leader possesses high motivation, drive, and persistence. Persuasiveness emerges as a pervasive characteristic. Other factors displayed by the leader are the ability to reconcile conflicting demands, structure expectations, and consider the follower's welfare. In summary, Stogdill drew the following composite picture of the leader.

> The leader is characterized by a strong desire for responsibility and task completion, vigor and persistence in the pursuit of goals, venturesomeness and originality in problem solving, drive to exercise initiative in social situations, self-confidence and sense of personal identity, willingness to accept consequences of decision and action, readiness to absorb interpersonal stress, willingness to tolerate frustration and delay, ability to influence other persons' behavior and capacity to structure social interaction systems to the purpose at hand.[43]

In conclusion, it must be emphasized that a wide variety of factors influence and contribute to the emergence, selection, preparation, and development of leaders. Among the factors that exert an influence are status and personality, intellectual capacity, the size, structure, and composition of the group of followers, the goals of the group, and other factors such as the setting, ie, the situation. Leaders are judged to be successful not on the possession of a combination of characteristics or traits, but rather on what they accomplish.

STATE OF LEADERSHIP IN NURSING

The state of leadership in nursing may be succinctly described as severely deficient both in quantity and quality. The current literature in nursing shows the lack of leadership within the field and pleads for nurses who can provide decisive leadership based upon knowledge. Higgs and Magill state:

> In these days of change and crisis nursing often bemoans a lack of leadership; our literature is replete with cries for leaders who will help us refine our roles and mold us into a cohesive force capable of influencing the direction in which health care systems develop.[44]

The issues in regard to leadership in nursing must be resolved by the profession. The health care and nursing requirements of the country are determined for the most part outside the field of nursing. But it is within organized nursing that the means for meeting the nursing needs must be devised. The top leadership in nursing today, as in the past, resides with administrators of nursing service institutions and education programs. Administrators of nursing services and education programs are the voices for the profession and the advocates of theory and practice in nursing. However, in the health care field, colleagues and peers castigate nursing administration as removing nurses from the client. The point must be made and accepted that in nursing there are various levels of leaders; every nurse must be a leader. There are leader practitioners, clinicians, head nurses, supervisors, directors, teachers, instructors, professors, and deans. The need for leadership is well known and documented within the profession and throughout the nation. The state of leadership will be examined by reviewing two major situations in the field, namely, nursing service and nursing education.

Nursing Service

There is a critical shortage of nurse leaders in nursing service. Leaders with political, behavioral, and social skills are required to develop nursing and health care focused on individual stylized comprehensive care for clients and families. The severe lack of quality practitioners with knowledge about theory and practice in leadership, who can utilize leadership ability to provide individualized care to clients, militates against the provision of quality health care. According to Haase and Smith:

> Nursing is an emerging profession. Expertise resides with the few. A role structure with meaning for the practitioners and the employing agency has yet to emerge. Utilization of nurses in many settings is misaligned with preparation for practice, highly developed nursing skills are unused, understandings weakened and new graduates co-opted into the unyielding bureaucratic structure of many hospitals.[45]

Nursing services within hospitals are notorious for their bureaucratic structure accompanied by strong authoritarianism that is a vestige of the development of nursing from the military hospital model. The founder of modern nursing, Florence Nightingale, made her impact on nursing care in the military setting during the Crimean War. Militarism is a curse upon nursing that endures. The bureaucratic setting and the authoritarianism of the institutions that employ most practitioners in the field limits and disqualifies nurses from leading peers, subordinates, and clients.

In the total situation of nursing service there is a negative feeling regarding leadership and positions for leaders. Most nurses express the desire to give direct care to people rather than to lead. Most are educated to give care that excludes the theory and practice of leadership. Nurses lack a sense of themselves as leaders and, unfortunately, few role models of leaders exist in the nursing service. Practitioners are devoid of the preparation to become leaders. Within nursing it is thought that leadership is something the nurse learns in practice when she becomes an administrator, or by happenstance, or that leading is an inborn or native ability. Negative feelings regarding leadership are reinforced by emphasis on and tributes to nurse practitioners and clinicians. Nurses who are practitioners will respect leadership if the recognized leaders in nursing, that is, educators, administrators, consultants, scholars, and researchers, respect leadership and insist upon it at all levels in the field. Staff nurses, head nurses, and supervisors in service agencies will respect and exert leadership if the recognized leaders respect leadership. Nurses will value leading theory, nursing theory—things of the mind and spirit—when, and if, society values them.

Other health care workers such as physicians are heard to say repeatedly, "We don't want chiefs, just nurses to care for our patients." Nursing administration and leadership have been denigrated by an insistence that leadership or the skills of administration be used to remove a nurse from the client's side. Such a restricted and narrow view fails to consider the fact that nursing is a service to people only in relationships with clients and that a large number of clients can be served well when leadership is utilized.

For years the hue and cry across the nation has been related to a shortage of bedside nurses for the care of ill, hospitalized clients, without concern for research and study of the problems and needs within nursing services. The reason physicians and others say they want a nurse to give care to patients is their limited view of the total health care needs of people and the role nurses can play in this care. Within the health professions, and in nursing in particular, an all-or-nothing attitude is still supported. An example of this attitude is that all nurses must be illness care practitioners, or specialized clinicians, or that all nurses must be at the patient's bedside, or that all must be administrators. Leadership in nursing will and must coexist and be utilized by all practitioners, be they clinicians, teachers, researchers, scholars, consultants, deans, or directors. Leadership is not the exclusive right or responsibility of persons in certain positions in nursing. As Young stated, "A profession cannot grow without a diversity of talent among its practitioners and without leadership to catalyze these talents." [46]

We need to develop leadership so that nurses can participate in the decision-making processes in primary care, community settings, clinical nursing, acute and chronic care settings, rehabilitation, and health services to persons of all ages, groups, and families. The leadership for nursing service in the variety of health care agencies of our nation has heretofore resided in the registered nurse who graduated from a hospital diploma nursing program. A high proportion of the nursing service administrative personnel within health care institutions are relatively senior and have not sought continuing or further preparation; their tenure in the position tends to be too short or too long. Therefore, role models of practitioners as leaders in nursing service are few and far between.

STATISTICS

The state of leadership is revealed by an analysis of the current statistics regarding nursing manpower. Since women predominate in nursing, a look at women in the labor force of our country is in order.

According to the April 1970 Statistical Bulletin from the Metropolitan Life Insurance Company, 22.4 million women aged 25 and over were reported as gainfully employed. This is an increase of almost one-fourth since 1960. The most rapid rise occurred among professional, technical, and kindred workers.

In 1970 nearly one-sixth of all employed women were employed as professional and kindred workers. It was also reported that over one-half of the women employed in the category of professional, technical, and kindred workers had a college education.[47] Women have increased their participation in the labor market with each successive census. Women have improved their educational attainment and this has been paralleled by their increased participation in the labor force outside the home.

Based on recent statistics, 1,127,647 registered nurses held licenses to practice in 1972; however, only 69 percent reported they were employed in nursing—a total of 778,470. Hospitals continue to be the major employers of registered nurses. In 1972, of all employed nurses, 64.2 percent worked in hospitals.[48]

The fact that the majority of employed licensed nurses are working in hospitals is very significant in relation to leadership. More than one-half of the nurses practicing today do so within an organizationally structured institution. Hospitals, as presently structured, limit a nurse's ability to develop and exert leadership. Within a hospital setting a nurse's power and authority are contingent entirely on the approval of physicians and hospital administrators. Limiting their power and authority diminishes the possibilites for implementing nursing leadership. Roberts and Group state: "It is increasingly evident that institutionally based nursing programs are probably one of the most deleterious elements in nursing today. The majority of nurses are working in and employed by hospitals, some of the worst military bureaucracies extant at the present time."[49]

The majority of nurses practicing today hold less than a baccalaureate degree. The baccalaureate degree program in nursing prepares the beginning professional nursing practitioner. In 1972, 81 percent of all employed registered nurses received their education either in a diploma program in nursing or through an associate degree program in nursing.[50] The diploma and the associate degree programs in nursing prepare technical nurses. Only 14.3 percent of employed registered nurses hold baccalaureate degrees and 3.4 percent hold graduate degrees.[51] An overwhelming number of nurses in the labor market have not completed the first level of professional nursing preparation. The number of practicing nurses with higher degrees is even less. There is a definitive, recognized shortage of educated administrative personnel for nursing in the United States. In 1972, 1.2 percent of nurses in hospital nursing services held masters degrees and 0.1 percent held doctoral degrees.[51] The statistics speak for themselves in regard to the state of leadership in nursing service.

To further complicate the state of leadership, nursing services are provided by others in concert with the registered nurse. Nursing care is given by a wide variety of workers other than nurses. The registered nurse is complemented and supplemented by other types of nursing personnel who need to be guided and led in the provision of health care. Nurses are responsible for the nature, kind, and quality of all nursing care that clients receive within health care agencies. Other personnel assigned nursing duties are licensed practical nurses, nurse aides, orderlies, attendants, home health aides, homemakers, ward clerks, and a myriad of other technical assistants. Registered nurses are required to assume the responsibility for the preparation and supervision of these auxiliary workers in nursing. The registered nurse must oversee the performance of practical nurses and other nonprofessional personnel who give certain aspects of total comprehensive nursing care. The number of nursing auxiliary workers continues to grow at a rapid rate. This increases the need for all registered nurses to be prepared as leaders.

In 1970, according to Health Resources Statistics, a survey of nursing personnel conducted by the United States Public Health Service and the American Hospital Association, found that 559,071 nursing aides, orderlies, and attendants were employed in hospitals. This number grew to 875,000 in 1972. Also reported was the fact that the total number of home health aides and homemakers increased from 2,300 in 1960 to 25,000 in 1972.[52] All supplementary and auxiliary personnel in nursing are the responsibility of registered nurses in the employing institutions or agencies. Nurses must act as leaders in nursing service regardless of administrative position. There is a very obvious dearth of educationally prepared nurses with the ability to supply convincing answers or even to point out directions toward solutions of the ever-increasing problems within the illness and health care system. Leadership is something you don't know you need until you don't have it. The sudden, rapid spurt of auxiliary workers in nursing requires an increase of nurse leaders. Quality nursing care and improved health care in the United States will be accomplished when individual practitioners, staff nurses, head nurses, supervisors, and directors are prepared to assume their respective leadership responsibilities in nursing service. Presently, nursing service settings reflect a severe lack of educationally prepared leaders on all levels. There is indeed a critical shortage of educationally prepared nurse leaders to provide quality nursing service. Leaders in nursing must be developed through nursing education.

Nursing Education

The highest priority for nurse leaders at this time, when the state of leadership is severely deficient in quantity and quality, lies in education. In the academic setting leaders are prepared for distribution throughout the multiple and varied activities that constitute the field. Educators of leaders must be prepared in leadership to serve as role models for future leaders. Clearly the overriding need of the nursing profession at this time is for nurses who can move the frontiers of nursing knowledge forward and provide decisive leadership based upon that knowledge.

All professions proclaim the need for persons prepared with graduate degrees to assume top level positions, to conduct research, and to provide scholarship within the particular discipline. Nursing is perhaps the most needy of all when one considers the dearth of persons prepared with further, advanced, or graduate education. The first nurse to earn a doctoral degree did so in 1927.[53] Nursing education entered the system of higher education in the United States at the start of the twentieth century. This is recent when compared to the professions of law and medicine, where higher education began centuries ago. Since the first nurse earned a doctoral degree, the number of nurses with doctoral degrees has grown slowly but steadily to the approximately 1,200 at present. When one considers the needs of nursing, the number of doctorally prepared nurses is infinitesimal. Higher education is expected to prepare leaders. Collegiate nursing programs were envisioned by early nurse leaders as the method whereby persons can be prepared for leadership positions in nursing. Nurses with advanced education and high level expertise are sorely needed to provide faculty for the development of quality educational programs to prepare superb products. John Gardner has said: "Only high ability and sound education equip a man for the continuous seeking of new solutions." [54]

The aim of the profession is to educate large numbers of quality nurses at the baccalaureate degree level in nursing as beginning leaders. The numbers of nurses being educated at the college level is larger than ever before.

In the 1973–1974 academic year enrollment in baccalaureate nursing programs was higher than for any other kind of nursing program. A total of 94,379 students were enrolled in baccalaureate degree programs in nursing.[55] This is a bright note in a rather bleak picture and portends a brighter future. The growth of leaders in nursing has been retarded by the diffuse and multiple programs utilized for the education of nurses. With a beginning increase in enrollments in baccalaureate degree programs in nursing, the profession has a more substantial foundation for the development of leaders. The further education of nurses in increased numbers at the masters and doctoral levels will provide a better chance of bringing nurses with creative talent and leadership ability to the top leadership positions.

Leadership is impossible without a framework of shared goals. The profession must ask itself if failure to prepare quality leaders in the past is a result of the fact that nursing theory is lacking in our nursing education programs. Nurse educators and nurses universally define nursing as a science and a practice, then proceed to disregard the science portion and concentrate solely on practice. The definition of nursing as a science and as a practice requires the support of a theoretical framework from which principles and practices can be derived. The crisis in nursing leadership is also a crisis in the development of nursing theory. Quality practitioners and leaders will emerge when nursing education concentrates on implementing theories of nursing. Without a conceptual framework for curricula and a theoretical base for practice, nurses will never be able to take their proper place as leaders in nursing and among other health professionals in the delivery of health care.

NURSING THEORY

Many people bridle at the notion of theory. This seems to be especially true of nurses. To theorize or work at the theoretical level are notions that connote the vague, esoteric, or nonsensical. In one sense, to be theoretical is to be unconcerned about the needs of persons being cared for by nurses. Nurses like to remind themselves that they are action oriented. The profession prefers to consider nurses as doers, not thinkers or theory developers. Nurses are educated to be practitioners not theoreticians.

A theory is intended to be the skeletal structure of nursing learned during the formal educational process and then fleshed out by nursing research and nursing practice to become the base for spawning new knowledge and improving existing practice. The theory of most immediate and compelling concern to the practitioner of nursing is that which provides structure and unity to the nursing process.[56]

The practitioner is concerned with testing hypotheses or hunches and observing the consequences on the persons affected. Practitioners of professional nursing deal with ideas different from those related to objects or things. Professional nurses are vitally involved with the immediate impact of their actions on the lives of people. This means the professional practitioner of nursing must be sensitive to values and to the moral dimensions of theories that guide practice. Theory is not an impersonal set of notions that can be denied or acknowledged, utilized or ignored, as a nurse sees fit. Nursing theory, which guides nursing practice, is directive. Theory determines how one relates to and serves the persons committed to the nurse's care.[56]

The relationship between theory and practice is as follows: A nursing action is guided by nursing theory which, in turn, entails moral responsibility on the part of the nurse. On every level of nursing practice theory development is required. The same, and even more so, is true in nursing education. Theory is necessary. It helps practitioners and educators determine what is important and relevant to what they are attempting to do. In a world where the generation of knowledge has literally run rampant (this is true in health care as it is elsewhere), practitioners and educators can be overwhelmed by the morass of information and conflicting ideas. Theory helps the nurse to make important and useful judgments about data and information. Theory helps organize and logically relate information and ideas so that practice has a clear direction and purpose. Theory is the yardstick against which nursing practice is measured and evaluated. If practice does not prove functional, the logic of the connection between theory and practice can be studied. Data based on theory can be reexamined to determine the measures needed to adjust the practice. Often the reexamination reveals that the breakdown lies in the human link between theory and practice, ie, the nursing practitioner. The knowledgeable practitioner, grounded in theory, does not consider the breakdown disastrous but rather finds a way to develop a new practice to implement the theory.[56]

It may be unnecessary, impossible, or undesirable to translate all theory into practice. The knowledge that practice is grounded in theory coupled with an understanding of how the theory originated, will broaden one's perspective, deepen one's insight, and anchor one's confidence. Theory enables the nurse to describe, explain, and predict what is being done. It can be claimed with assurance that a nurse grounded in theory about man, society, health, and nursing will have a sense of stability and security that will enhance practice and improve capabilities of discharging the profound responsibility assumed when nursing and the preparation of nurses are the goals.

Perhaps in no field of endeavor have more mindless comments been made about theory than in the discipline of nursing. One constantly hears such statements as, "Don't bother me with your theories, I need something practical to take care of these patients." Of course, practicalities are required. But on what is nursing practice and care based? The answer is knowledge and theory. Such assertions are to be viewed as sad commentaries on the nurse educators who prepare nurse practitioners. Nursing education will fail to prepare quality nurse leaders until the theory of nursing practice is stressed in nursing education.

STATISTICS

Statistics of particular concern to the present state of leadership in nursing education are found in the 1974 NLN Nurse-Faculty Census. In January, 1974 an estimated total of 24,178 full-time and 5017 part-time nurse-faculty members were reported employed in all nursing education programs. In addition, there were 1139 unfilled budgeted positions among faculties of the nation's nursing schools. These estimates were based on responses from 2652 schools of all types: 319 baccalaureate and higher degree, 565 associate degree, 491 diploma, and 1277 practical nursing programs.[57] The unfilled, budgeted, position figures do not include positions needed but not budgeted because of financial restrictions. The unfilled budgeted positions are extremely cogent because they reveal a major problem in nursing. An extreme shortage exists for those faculty qualified by education and experience to teach in the nation's nursing schools where leaders for the profession are prepared.

Another important set of statistics is the data related to educational preparation of the faculty who serve as role models of leadership and who prepare the leaders. A considerable majority of full-time faculty members had earned at least a baccalaureate degree. However, the baccalaureate degree program in nursing prepares a generalist practitioner, not a teacher. All preparation for specialization in nursing takes place at the masters degree level, which prepares teachers, clinicians, researchers, consultants, and nursing service administrators. The educational attainment of faculties in nursing is a rather dismal picture since the highest earned credentials of all faculty in the 1974 Faculty Census were as follows: doctorate, 2.9 percent; masters, 43.7 percent; baccalaureate, 38.3 percent; associate degree, 1.6 percent; and diploma 13.5 percent.[57] More than one-half of the faculty in the nursing schools of the nation do not possess the credentials required to be considered educationally qualified for teaching. Hence there is a tremendous need for further academic preparation among the faculties in nursing schools.

What are the statistics in relation to the nursing schools where potential leaders will be prepared? The most up-to-date figures for numbers of programs in nursing that prepare students to take licensing examinations in order to practice nursing are as follows in the year 1975: associate degree, 604, diploma, 495, and baccalaureate, 316.[58] The total number of programs that purport to prepare leaders of nursing is only 21 percent of the total. There has been an increase in the number of nursing programs at the associate degree, baccalaureate, masters, and doctoral degree levels. There are 86 masters degree programs and 8 doctoral programs in nursing.[59,60]

It seems evident that the major problem in the state of leadership in nursing is the overwhelming need for educationally qualified persons steeped in nursing theory. The need for nurses prepared at the masters and doctoral levels is tremendous. The highest priority of need is in academia. The educational programs can only prepare qualified practitioners for leadership if the faculties in the programs are qualified. Secondly, and equally important, is the need for nurses with graduate preparation in nursing for the service agencies that provide direct health care to the public. Doctorally prepared people are required to fill strategic positions of importance in the profession in consultation, research, and policy formation of health and nursing care at the local, state, regional, and national levels. As stated by Leininger:

> In sum, this is a highly challenging, changing and critical period for nurse leaders in academia and service settings. Large scale and complex organizations, political regimes, professional competition, unit leadership, societal attitudes, interdisciplinary pressures, limited finances and space and the need for major changes in health care all are challenging nurses and nurse leaders. These challenges are before us at a time when there is a critical shortage of strong, competent, politically astute nurse leaders.[61]

Concepts and theories related to leadership will be explored in Chapter 2.

References

1. Stogdill RM: Handbook of Leadership—A Survey of Theory and Research. New York, The Free Press, 1974, p 7.
2. Drucker PF: The Effective Executive. New York, Harper & Row, 1967.
3. *Idem:* p viii.
4. *Idem:* p 111.

5. *Idem:* p 111-112.
6. Stogdill RM: Handbook of Leadership—A Survey of Theory and Research. New York, The Free Press, p viii.
7. Weisner J: Time, July 15, 1974, p 23.
8. Morris R: Time, July 15, 1974, p 23.
9. *Idem:* p 24.
10. Levison H: The Exceptional Executive. Cambridge, Mass., Harvard University Press, 1968, p 95.
11. *Idem:* p 49.
12. Drucker PF: The Effective Executive. New York, Harper & Row, 1967, p 91.
13. Russell F: The Shadow of Blooming Grove. New York, McGraw-Hill Book Co, 1968, p 477.
14. Shannon WV: The American Irish. New York, Collier Books, 1966, p 119.
15. Levison H: The Exceptional Executive. Cambridge, Mass, Harvard University Press, p 16.
16. Miller M: Plain Speaking. New York, Berkley Medallion Books, 1974, p 231.
17. Higgs Z, Magill KA: Nursing Leadership—needed for our transitional times. NY State Nurs Assoc 5:20-24, 1974.
18. Miller DI: Education for Nursing Service Administration. Nurs Forum 7:375-385, 1968.
19. Kron T: The Management of Patient Care. Philadelphia, WB Saunders Co, 1971, p 45.
20. Kelly DM: Musings on leadership. Superv Nurse 3:5, Dec 1972.
21. *Idem*
22. Eggers ET: The essence of leadership. Superv Nurse 3:23-27, Dec 1972.
23. Meleis AI, Farrell K: Operation concern—a study of senior nursing students in three nursing programs. Nurs Res 23:461-468, 1974.
24. Fleishman EA: Manual for Leadership Opinion Questionnaire. Chicago, Science Research Associates, 1969.
25. Gruenfeld L and Kassum S: Supervisory style and organizational effectiveness in a pediatric hospital. Personnel Psychol 26:531-544, 1973.
26. Kelly W: Psychological prediction of leadership in nursing. Nurs Res 23:38-42, 1974.
27. Lukens LG: Personality patterns and choice of clinical nursing specialization. Nurs Res 14:210-221, 1965.
28. Gilbert MA: Personality profiles and leadership potential of medical-surgical and psychiatric nursing graduate students. Nurs Res 24:125-130, 1975.

29. Maslow AH: The Farther Reaches of Human Nature, Chap 18. New York, The Viking Press, 1971, pp 239-248.
30. *Idem:* p 241.
31. *Idem:* p 242.
32. Sirota D, Wolfson AD: Pragmatic approach to people problems: Harv Bus Rev 51:120-128, 1973.
33. Stogdill RM: Handbook of Leadership—A Survey of Theory and Research. New York, The Free Press, p 23.
34. Leadership for improving instruction, 1960 Yearbook. Washington, Association for Supervision and Curriculum Development, 1960, p 182.
35. New Jersey Bell Telephone Company; Tele-news Release, Aug 1975.
36. Stogdill RM: Handbook of Leadership—A Survey of Theory and Research. New York, The Free Press, p 76.
37. *Idem:* p 77.
38. Time Inc.: The Sexes, May 26, 1975. New York, pp 40-41.
39. *Idem:* pp 40-41.
40. National Student Nurse Association: NSNA News, June 1975, New York, pp 8-9.
41. Stogdill RM: Handbook of Leadership—A Survey of Theory and Research. New York, The Free Press, p 78.
42. *Idem:* p 80.
43. *Idem:* p 81.
44. Higgs Z, Magill KA: Nursing Leadership—needed for our transitional times. NY State Nurs Assoc 5:20, 1974.
45. Haase P, Smith M: Nursing Education in the South 1973. Pathways to Practice. Vol 1. Atlanta, Southern Regional Education Board, 1973, p 3.
46. Young L: Room at the top: a place for nurse administrators. J Nurs Administr 20:85, Nov-Dec 1972.
47. Metropolitan Life: Statistical Bulletin, Nov, 1974, p. 8.
48. American Nurses Association. Facts About Nursing 72-73. Kansas City, 1974, p 6.
49. Roberts J, Group T: The women's movement and nursing. Nurs Forum 12:3, 1973, p 320.
50. Facts About Nursing 72-73. Kansas City, 1974, p 7.
51. *Idem:* p 10.
52. US Department of Health, Education, and Welfare: Health resources statistics 1972-1973. Washington DC, p 215.
53. American Nurses Foundation: International Directory of Nurses with Doctoral Degrees. Kansas City, 1973, p v.
54. Gardner J: Excellence. New York, Harper Brothers, 1961, p 35.

55. Ozimek D: The Future of Nursing Education. New York, National League for Nursing, 1975, p 14.
56. Thompson L: The nature and need of theory. Educ Forum 39:473-477, 1975.
57. National League for Nursing: 1974 NLN Nurse Faculty Census. New York, 1975, National League for Nursing.
58. National League for Nursing: 1975 State Approved Schools of Nursing-RN. New York, 1975, p 114.
59. National League for Nursing: Some Statistics on Baccalaureate and Higher Degree Programs in Nursing 1973-74. New York, 1975, p 3.
60. *Idem:* p 1.
61. Leininger M: The leadership crisis in nursing: a critical problem and challenge. J Nurs Administr 40:34, Mar-Apr 1974.

CHAPTER 2
Concepts and Theories Related to Leadership

As used in the literature, the terms leader, supervisor, manager, and executive as well as leadership, authority, organization, influence, and power are used interchangeably. It is not surprising to find an article entitled leadership devoted solely to management, the manager, and the goals of the formal organization, with almost no mention of leadership except for the title.

In this text, leadership is viewed as a concept in itself, permeating all human associations and distinct from formal and informal organizations and hierarchical arrangements. Leadership can be seen in action wherever a person, designated the leader, is involved with one or more persons who are willing to be influenced in goal setting and achievement.

AUTHORITY, POWER, AND INFLUENCE

There are three terms that have an impact, a relationship, or that are used in conjunction with leadership—authority, power, and influence. It is important to define these terms and distinguish their use

Concepts and Theories Related to Leadership   39

in relation to leadership. These terms are often used interchangeably, resulting in misuse and misunderstanding, contributing to the confusion surrounding the concept of leadership. Webster supports this by including influence and power as synonyms for authority.[1] Authority is defined as "the power or right to give commands, enforce obedience; the power or influence resulting from knowledge, prestige; a person with much knowledge or experience in some field, whose opinion is considered expert." [2]

Influence is defined as the power of persons or things to affect others, seen only in its effects—the power of a person or group to produce effects without exercising physical force or authority, based on wealth, social position, and ability. Influence implies the power of persons or things to affect others. Authority implies the power to command acceptance, belief, and obedience based on strength of character and expert knowledge. Prestige implies the power to command esteem and admiration.[3]

In yet another dictionary, power is considered to be a latent or inherent property of a person, capable of bringing about moral or physical changes—one who experiences great influence.[4] Authority means legal power, the right to command or act, power and influence of character or office.

We intend to explore the theoretical considerations for terms or concepts of authority, power, and influence that have been developed by various authors to enlighten nursing educators and practitioners to the dimensions of nursing leadership behavior and to serve to make the available research more meaningful. This theoretical framework may guide future research and practice relating to nursing leadership behavior with the hope that a basic, systematic, theoretical framework will emerge that will be acceptable, useful, and workable for the development of leadership potential for the nurse leaders "to be" and to support and enhance the development of recognized nurse leaders.

Many authors have thought or speculated about, researched, and analyzed one or more of these terms. Duncan, Professor of Education at Ohio State University, has usefully clarified the concepts of authority, power, and influence, which he considers are three basic leadership relations.[5] His presentation is directly applicable to nursing, since interpersonal encounters with clients (individuals, families, groups), peers, and colleagues are emphasized. He believes that authority, power, and influence are basic, interrelated, intertwined, and enmeshed, but that distinguishable relationships exist between the leader and those who are led.[6] To the casual observer authority, power, and influence would appear to be the same. Duncan supports the need to distinguish among these terms and the implied relationship between them to promote the analysis and understanding of behaviors which collectively make up a significant portion of the functions of the leader with respect to those he is leading.[6]

Authority

Authority is defined by Duncan as "an interpersonal relationship in which one person is given the right to make selected decisions that affect another's behavior."[7] He further explains that the right to make decisions affecting another person derives from common and statutory law and such extralegal realities as cultural and institutional norms. It can be assumed that one has authority when his right to make decisions affecting other people's behavior goes unchallenged; authority may be questioned when the right to make a decision is challenged.[8]

Merton pointed out that leadership as a mode of social influence is not the same as authority, which is an attribute of a social position. He uses examples of the judge, the organizational executive, the foreman, and the head nurse as having authority by virtue of the positions they hold. It must be emphasized that they may or may not also exert leadership. He states that "authority involves the legitimated rights of a position that require others to obey. . . ." He contrasts this with his belief that "leadership is an interpersonal relation in which others comply because they want to, not because they have to." He goes on to say that leadership can be found at every level of an organization and that leaders and influential persons sometimes hold formal offices of authority but sometimes do not. A distinction between authority and leadership must be made in order to understand problems related to authority and leadership and why some persons in positions of authority are more effective than others.[9]

Bennis believes that authority is abrogated by those who simply maintain role incumbency and, on the other hand, by the role occupant with technical competence and expertise. He differentiates two elements for technical competence: (a) knowledge of performance criteria, such as production and marketing, and (b) knowledge of the human aspects of administration, such as coordination and communication. Bennis quotes Secretary of State Kissinger as stating that due to the complexity, size, and interdependency of unity of organizations, knowledge of purpose and knowledge of administration are required of contemporary executives.[10]

Dalton, Barnes, and Zaleznik state that it is widely accepted that authority exists only when compliance with directives occurs, and that it is the accepted right to direct and alter behavior held as a general value judgment in the minds of those who initiate or act upon directives. "Directive" is used broadly to encompass written or verbal means of expressing direction for other people's behavior. They believe the concept of authority in formal organizations is more specifically the intended direction and content of influence. Whether or not attempts to influence are completely successful, the significance of formal organization and its prescribed patterns of influence do not diminish. The significance of formal organization as an input affecting thought and action does not diminish, but even if most individuals would not follow the prescribed pattern completely, they would respond to influence not encompassed in the structure.[11]

Looking at the formal organization structure, Dalton et al view authority as the prescribed expectations that one individual should exert control and direction over other individuals within defined areas of competence.[12] Authority is considered to be a structural variable, initially external to individuals comprising the organization. Through the process of influence (which is the use of authority to alter behavior), a latent attribute of the organization structure is converted into a manifest demand from one person to others on expected action. "What stands between authority as a structural variable and influence is an outcome of interpersonal events concerning the work which goes on within individuals in response to the authority in the structure, or its intended uses to affect behavior." [13]

In terms of the structure of authority, it is believed that it could take many forms and is subject to alteration and that the obligation and right to create or change an authority structure are basic to the core authority relationships:

> The traditional concept of authority with its emphasis on voluntary compliance leaves a large gap between authority as a structural variable and influence as actual direction or behavior. This gap is not closed satisfactorily by noting that influence occurs in ways other than compliance to directives as . . . in coercion and persuasion.[14]

Dalton et al go further and point out that a person anticipates that he will receive direction from persons designated as superiors in the organizational hierarchy when he joins the organization. They believe that, in addition to being a quantitative variable, authority is comprised of elements related to job responsibilities and areas of competence (positional and professional authority). Positional authority arises from implicit or explicit agreement among members of an organization to designate the rights of individuals to direct the activities of others as prescribed. Professional authority arises from the needs of the formal organization for the application of specialized knowledge and expertise gained through education.[15]

Barnard previously described authority along two dimensions —authority of position held by virtue of his formal position in the organizational hierarchy and authority of leadership based on superior ability, knowledge, and understanding, regardless of formal position.[16]

It must be obvious that although there is no consensus as to how the term authority should be used, related elements emerge when a variety of definitions and descriptions are compiled. The effective utilization of professional expertise, viewed as the second base of authority, should result in the solution of problems and successful adaptation to the environment.[17] But Thompson points out cogently that the most symptomatic characteristic of modern bureaucracy is the growing imbalance between ability and authority.[18] This can certainly be as true for some health organizations as for formal bureaucratic organizations.

Kalisch has a scholarly treatise on Aesculapian authority in which she describes the remarkable power the physician wields. He holds practically all control in the illness care environment. "This authority is utilized to convince patients that they are indeed sick, and, furthermore, they must submit to various treatments, hospitalization, and curtailment of normal activities." [19]

She draws upon Paterson's analysis of Aesculapian authority, which combines three different kinds of authority to account for its extreme potency. First, the physician carries the authority of an expert, as is true of all people who have the knowledge and skills essential for rendering a needed service valued by society. Second, part of this superpower is morally based, having been derived from the Hippocratic oath. It gives the physician the right to control the patient because he is believed to be morally committed to act for the good of his patients. He is a professional, guided by certain ethical principles, and thus is believed to act in the clients' interest rather than his own. The thought that he might not do his very best never occurs to most people. Third, and perhaps most significant, is the result of tradition that dates back centuries to when medicine was a product of natural philosophy. This power stems from the concept that the physician has license to control by reason of God-given graces. People believe in a vague and almost unconscious way that the physician has special connections with the world of the unknown, philosophically and spiritually.[19]

Tannenbaum, Weschler, and Massarik propose that although authority is commonly viewed as originating at the top of an organizational hierarchy, flowing downward by virtue of delegation, this is formal and not necessarily effective authority. The acceptance of authority by those subject to it transforms formal or nominal authority to real authority. Tannenbaum et al define authority as an interpersonal relationship in which a person (the subordinate) accepts a decision that directly affects his behavior, which is made by a person viewed as the superior.[20] Thus, it is the subordinate or recipient who decides to accept or reject such a decision. Acceptance implies granting authority. The hierarchic focus is evident, but giving authority rests at the lower hierarchic levels. Tannenbaum et al explain why an individual would accept given authority. Generally, the advantages to the person who is subordinate outweigh the disadvantages. The advantages are that an individual: (a) can contribute to the attainment of the enterprise purpose recognized as being good; (b) may attain approbation of co-workers; (c) can obtain rewards from his superior; (d) can act in accordance with his own moral standards; (e) can avoid the necessity of accepting responsibility; (f) may be responding to such qualities of his superior as age, superior ability or experience, character, reputation, and personality.[21]

Acceptance of authority should be a free choice. "When an individual is forced by another to do something against his will, coercion is involved. Coercion is a behavioral manifestation in which thoughts and actions of a person or a group are compelled or restrained by another." [22]

Turning to the academic setting, Clark studied faculty organization and authority and noted the difference in authority based on broad changes in the nature of the campus. Authority is felt to be conditioned by the nature of the work, the technology of the organization, and by the patterns of status that prevail as well as by traditional sentiments.[23] He points out that the large college or university cannot remain as unitary as the small one. Authority must be extensively delegated and subsidiary units formed around many centers of authority. The subunits formed stem from a plurality of purpose, indicating that movement has been from single- to multipurpose colleges.[24] The campus tends toward composite structure, a multiplicity of subcultures, intense professionalism, and some bureaucratic coordination. Changes in faculty organization and authority accommodate these trends by segmentation, by federated professionalism, and by the growth of individual power centers.

The decision-making power and influence of the faculty is now more segmented by subcollege, division, and, particularly, department. The authority of the faculty, which flows out toward departments and other units, becomes located in the hands of highly specialized experts, and takes on some characteristics of professional authority. Professional and bureaucratic authority are both necessary, for each performs an essential function—professional authority protects the exercise of the special expertise of the technologist allow-

Concepts and Theories Related to Leadership   45

ing his judgment to be preeminent in many matters. Bureaucratic authority functions to coordinate the work of technologists with other major elements of the university.²⁵

Bureaucratic direction is not capable of providing certain expert judgments; professional direction is not capable of providing overall coordination. The problem of allocating authority between professionals and bureaucrats varies in intensity and form in different kinds of organizations. Where professional influence is high and there is one dominant professional group, the organization will be integrated by the imposition of professional standards; where professional influence is high and there are a number of professional groups, the organization will be split by professionalism. The personal authority of the experts varies widely with the establishment, and often with rank and seniority. The campus is a place where strong forces cause the growth of some individuals into centers of power. The technical nature of specialized lines of work of most academic persons is a source of personal authority. The personal authority of some professional experts is greatly enhanced by money. The power of the individual faculty member is going up while the power of the collective faculty is going down because the individual as researcher, scholar, and consultant relates increasingly to grant-giving agencies of the federal government and to foundations.²⁶

A direct relation of faculty members to external sources of support affects the distribution of influence within the campus, redistributing influence from those who do not have such contacts to those who do, and moving power from the faculty as a whole and as smaller collectives to individual professors. The source of great influence in the modern American university is less internal and less tied to particular positives. It is more external and more tied to national and international prestige in a discipline and to contact with support for research and scholarship.²⁷

Personal authority of the professional expert is increased in our time by the competitiveness of the job market.²⁸ "Expertise is the dominant characteristic of the campus and organization and authority cluster around it. . . . The faculty moves toward a decentralized or federated structure, and authority moves toward clusters of experts and the individual expert. Thus, professional authority tends to become dominant and collegiate and bureaucratic features fall into subsidiary places." [29]

In his study of the influences of administrative structure of American colleges and universities on academic work, Blau indicates that bureaucratic authority has its source in a superior official position, which bestows the power to command on incumbents and includes sanctions needed to enforce these commands. On the other hand, professional authority has its source in expert knowledge resulting from prolonged specialized education, allowing those who possess this knowledge and expertise to direct the endeavors of others to achieve certain ends.[30]

Although educating students is the professional responsibility of the faculty, one needs only to determine the degree to which educational decisions are centralized in a university to determine if the university conforms to the bureaucratic model rather than to the professional model.[31]

The power acquired in social exchange by faculties who have superior academic standing is the source of their authority within the university or college rather than reliable performance of their duties. Scientists and scholars who command wide respect among colleagues in their discipline achieve influential positions outside their own academic institution, are sought after by other institutions, and are needed by their own, since its academic standing depends on them. "It has been demonstrated that research has more prestige than teaching in academic circles with the result that research faculties consequently have more influence in their institution than teaching faculties." [32]

Influence accrued by a university faculty with high academic standing becomes institutionalized in the form of faculty authority enhancing the influence of individual faculty members, regardless of their personal academic standing. Centralized control is reduced by a faculty government in a college or university which, in turn, strengthens the authority of the faculty in a university or college. "Power institutionalized in the form of authority endures and becomes independent of the original source of power." [33] The great financial resources of large universities gives those controlling them, namely, the Board of Trustees and central administration, much power. Since control over the allocation of economic resources is the ultimate source of power in an institution, it can be said that the basic power in major universities is exercised by the Board of Trustees and the central administration, in spite of the extensive decentralization of authority over academic affairs to the faculty.[33]

To summarize, there are varied dimensions of the term authority. There are also two major types of authority upon which power relations develop; these are hierarchic authority, which vests power or its potential in an organization, and professional authority, which involves educational and experiential expertise. These dimensions are supported by Clark and Blau who studied authority in an academic setting.

For influence to occur in hierarchic formal organizations, members must recognize and be willing to accept influence from above.[34] The military services are probably the best example of authoritarian hierarchic relationships, but the medical profession has, until very recently, maintained an authoritarian set of hierarchic relationships, particularly with respect to relations between doctors, nurses, and paraprofessionals.[35]

Duncan makes an interesting point when he says that the regular exercise of authority is essential to its preservation. Duncan's definition of an authority relationship focuses on an interpersonal relationship in which one person is given the right to make selected decisions that affect another's behavior. This interpersonal position is supported by Tannenbaum et al except for their focus on a superior–subordinate relationship as an additional dimension.

Power

The second term of significance is power. Power is readily apparent in conversations today, with concern centered on the uses and abuses of power. This portion of the chapter will focus on power as a concept and will review significant developments and the composition of power as proposed by authorities. Again, Duncan is a valuable source to distinguish the difference between power and authority. He views these two terms as complementary yet different and distinguishable. "Power is defined as an interpersonal relationship in which one person is capable of satisfying or not satisfying the needs of another person and, as a result, is capable of affecting the other person's behavior." [36] Involved in the exercise of power are the satisfaction and denial of need fulfillment of another person or group. Duncan explains that, as used in our society, power relies heavily upon psychologic conditions of human experience. There is no doubt that we have many physiologic needs, but the needs more readily satisfied or denied are those of a psychologic nature. Thus, power has a positive and a negative dimension, ie, positive where needs are satisfied and negative where needs are not satisfied.

He distinguishes between the exercise of authority as the exercise of an orderly rule of law through decision making affecting people's behavior and the exercise of power as the manipulation of conditions related to satisfying or not a person's physiologic or psychologic needs, thus affecting his behavior. Authority and power are not only complementary but often are exercised together. However, the capacity of authority or power to affect human behavior is derived from different requirements in human social conditions. Authority relationships are established in society to ensure that an orderly process of decision making can take place to benefit all citizens. The development of power relations occurs in society as the physiologic and psychologic needs of people become manifest and are expressed in human behavior.[37]

From the point of view of formal organizations, Dalton et al suggest that the silent work which ensues within individuals is the variable intervening between the input of structural change and the outcome of interaction, performance, and productivity. Power is one dimension of this intervening variable and is distinguished from authority and influence.[38] Power is defined as the potential a person has to guide, direct, control, or alter the behavior of others with the amount of power differing with individuals. This difference is evident. It depends on how a person in the organization can bring together authority stemming from his hierarchic location in the formal organization and is made personal by assessment of self and goals as a member of a particular organization. Another facet in the variability of power is seen in the person who may have considerable authority but may not wish to or may be unable to use this authority, resulting in little power or a low potential to affect the thought and actions of others. Low power can result when an individual has little authority related to formal organization, even though he is highly motivated to act and influence others.[39] Dalton and Barnes believe the crux of power is what goes on between people rather than within an individual, and the terms power and authority are attributes of the relationship rather than the individual.[40] This view is a contrast to Zaleznik's belief that power is established when individuals internalize what is external and an attribute of structure and that one's power is subject to increases and decreases, depending on the holder's success in influencing others.[41]

Other dimensions of power revealed by Dalton et al include that in which affecting outcomes in any sphere of human activity involves individuals in using themselves. Self-assertions express power, and unless one visualizes only passive persons, the notion of power, the basis upon which it is established, and how it is used, becomes an important variables in all human sciences, particularly in organization and management.[42] The particular mode of synthesis of both professional and positional authority depends upon the individual's style of work and the way he develops power. Although efforts to rationalize organizations lean heavily on the ascendancy of professional authority—often at the expense of positional authority—it may be possible for positional authority to resume a primary position. "As specialists get promotions, for example, they move upward in the hierarchy and away from specific applications of knowledge and technique. This trend may be expressed as the movement from specialist to generalist or from staff to line work." [43]

In the formal organization the crucial issue affecting power is the relative distribution of authority, since no absolute measures of authority are being subjected to comparisons of gains or losses in the proportion allocated. This is the distinction between absolute and relative amounts of power and authority.[44]

Based on research, certain predictable behaviors have been found to occur when there is a conflict of interest among individuals who have power. Behavioral alternatives include: (a) seeking to enhance one's power in responding to change through coalition formation; (b) bargaining—negotiation of obvious conflict will become evident with or without coalition; (c) leaving by those in a condition of deprivation if bargaining is ineffective; (d) adjusting to lessened authority and power if alternative positions outside the organization are unavailable or too difficult to secure.[45]

Still another dimension of power is the ability to induce change. The application of this dimension is related to authority and influence. The power to induce change is inherent in the authority of formal position, support of superiors and subordinates, and also the reputation of the person for goal achievement.[46]

Griffiths indicates that power is sought in order to control the decision-making process in an organization. This is readily apparent in the world of business and politics and somewhat less apparent in the world of education. Power is viewed as a function of the decision made. A person has power to the extent that his decisions affect the course of action of an enterprise to a greater degree than do decisions made by others and that his decisions influence other decisions.[47]

Tannenbaum et al caution that the concept of power frequently connotes a potential for coercion based upon such factors as physical force, informal social pressure, law, and authority. Actually, a leader has available power derived from the mentioned external sources as well as from such inner resources as understanding and flexibility.[48]

Power is regarded by Stogdill as a form of influence relationship whereas social power is defined as an influence relationship between persons. All sources of power yield influence, with the leader drawing (consciously and unconsciously) upon multiple sources of power in the real sense. "Reward and coercive power are probably the sources most easily manipulated by the leader." [49] The person who holds power has the advantage, but for every source of power, followers can use countermeasures to reduce the extent to which they are subject to influence. Stogdill believes that social power implies a relationship in which participants are bound together by interdependency, influence, and exchange. Failure to honor this mutual obligation results in a lack of a stable basis for the exercise of power. In a review of the research literature related to power, sources of power such as expertise, reference (liking), legitimation, coercion, and reward have been studied extensively. Stogdill concludes that power is but one aspect of role differentiation and is not synonymous with leadership.[50]

In another study of power, authority, and influence as they relate to organization, Aiken and Mott show that: (a) social power is potential energy created in the actual process of organizing or pooling usable individual energies—the usable and socially valued latent energy locked in human organization; (b) authority is consent legitimately given to groups or individuals to direct certain activities and to use certain resources to achieve collective purposes; (c) social influence is the attempt to utilize the energies of others to achieve a desired objective—it is action and it is social.[51] "Influencing and self-adjustment are major dynamic links between social power and authority on one hand and social control on the other. If control is the achievement of order, influencing includes those attempts to achieve it; social control is a product of many forces, successful influencing is one of them."[51]

Position, reputation, and personal traits are believed, by Aiken and Mott, to be primary determinants of the total amount of power to which a person or a group has access and can wield. Positional power signifies the maximum amount of power that could be utilized by virtue of one's position in an organization. Reputation for power can give its possessor access to power in a fashion similar to personal traits. "A person may be without a significant positional base for power, but still have great access to power because of the brilliance of his ideas, his knowledge of people and organization, or his persuasive abilities."[52] Thus, this person achieves access to power indirectly by influencing persons with positional power. A useful example is given when these authors note the importance of a person's reputation and skill in the strategy of bidding and bluffing in poker so that he wins even though he holds cards (resources) of less value than those of other players.[53]

Within an organization there is greater access to power when connective links are controlled, such as control of individuals or groups through whom communications must be made. Power is not viewed as energy directed in and of itself, but as latent energy to be taken into account by those who need or value it, accommodating or adjusting their actions to the fact it exists. "Decisions may be shaped by the perceived attitudes and aspirations of specific persons who are not actually involved in decision making and they may also be shaped by predominant values, norms, customs, or traditions. This power need not reside primarily in the decision-making structure."[54]

Authorization or the process of granting authority is related to social power in that it allocates power for selected purposes. Aiken and Mott view influencing and self-adjustment or accommodation as major links between social power and social control. They conclude that: (a) as the ratio of a specific group's power to the power of all groups in the organization increases, so does the social control achieved by this specific group; (b) as this social control ratio increases, the social control resulting from self-adjusting behavior by others will increase directly. However, the frequency of attempts at influencing may or may not increase; (c) as the ratio of influence attempts increase, the proportion of successful attempts to influence will increase directly.[55]

Hawley and Wirt in *The Search for Community Power* note that power can be seen as inherent fundamentally in institutions rather than in people and it can be viewed as a result of interpersonal relationships. What seems to be common to all views of power is a relationship between persons, one inducing another to do the former's will. They state that potential power is relatively unimportant until it is translated into interpersonal action to achieve compliance.[56]

According to Blau, formal organizations make power liquid by transforming the potential power of financial resources into actual power over employees, dependent on their incomes and by vesting this power in the form of institutional authority in official positions. "Since both financial resources and official authority reside in the formal organization and do not belong to its particular members, the power emanating from them can readily be transferred from existing personnel to replacements and from one position to another. Indeed the entire power of an organization may be transferred to enhance another, as illustrated by mergers of companies. . . . ."[57] Blau points out that the hierarchy of power facilitates the limited power of many lower managers to be accumulated through the chain of command into the controlling power of top executives. Thus, organizational power is viewed as more liquid than personal power due to the fact that the former can be accumulated as well as transferred.[57]

Etzioni defines organizational control structure as a distribution of means used by an organization to elicit performances it needs and to ascertain whether the quantities and qualities of these performances are in accord with organizational specifications. Organizations are unlike social units, such as the family and community, which have structure and control their members. Organizations have a distinct structure, but their problem of control is acute. Organizations' intense concern is performance; their tendency to be larger than natural units makes formal control mandatory. "Most organizations cannot rely on most of their participants to carry out assignments voluntarily, ie, to internalize their obligations."[58] Organizational members need supervision; supervisors also need supervision by persons who themselves are supervised.

Controls inherent in various organizational positions are categorized as physical, material, and symbolic. Physical controls, such as locks and the threat and use of physical means are called coercive power. Utilitarian power is derived from the use of material means, such as rewards of goods and services. The use of symbols (prestige, esteem, love, and acceptance) is termed identitive power. Identitive power generates more commitment than does utilitarian power, while coercive power is more alienating to those subject to it; ". . . the application of symbolic means of control tends to convince people; that of material means tends to build-up their self-oriented interests in conforming; and the use of physical means forces them to comply (as when a lock makes an inmate stay indoors)."[59] Organizations use more than one kind of power and tend to use fewer alienating means to control their higher than to control their lower ranks.

There is a significant difference in the degree to which control is needed in organizations because of differences in the degree of selection and socialization. The more selective organizations tend to be, the more effective they will be in carrying out their goals and the more efficient in cost per unit of output. The amount of control needed to attain a given level of effectiveness is lower when selectivity and socialization are both higher, and higher when both these dimensions are lower. The degree to which an organization selects its participants affects its need for controls in terms of the amount of resources and effort that must be invested to maintain the level of control considered adequate. Note the differences between and among organizations where coercion is dominant (concentration camp, prison), organizations where utilitarian power is dominant (factories, banks, insurance companies), and those where indentitive power dominates (colleges and universities, religious organizations, schools).[60]

The power used by an organization to control its participants is derived either from specific positions, personal qualities, or a combination of both. Personal power is almost always identitive power, based on the manipulation of symbols; this generates a commitment to the person who commands it, whereas positional power may be identitive, coercive, or utilitarian. Two spheres of activity open to control by organizations are those instrumental in dealing with input into the organization and the distribution of control within it. Activities that affect interpersonal relations within the organization and adherence to norms by participants are termed expressive.[61]

Dimensions of authority, power, and influence reflected in the academic setting were studied by a number of authors and common viewpoints as well as variations of those already presented were demonstrated. Lindquist and Blackburn report that governing as well as power researchers have generally developed four methodologies: (a) the structuralist—inventories the rank of persons who hold high positions in the collegiate and bureaucratic pyramids of campus decision making; (b) the reputationist—seeks to go beyond a description of governing structure and visible divison of labor by recording the perceptions of power held by campus members; (c) the decisionist—relies on observation or case history documentation of specific governance events; (d) the normative—determines the locus of campus power by identifying prevailing norms and values and persons they favor.[62]

Although there are limitations to each of these approaches, a combination of them has substantive merit and represents a methodology in itself. This methodology—the analysis of one or more institutions of the historic development of norms, values, decision-making structure, the division of labor, the history of decision making, plus the analysis of answers to questions about perceived power—was utilized by Lindquist and Blackburn. Although their results were based on an analysis of campus governance in one large state university throughout one academic year, the following conclusions were drawn and could be applicable in a broader context: (a) the holders of power in the university were the long-tenured, personally and professionally esteemed, experienced in local governance; the opinion leaders on campus issues; members of major governance councils; executive administrators or full professors; persons who are moderately open and democratic, but who respect both the legitimacy of administrative authority and the professional autonomy of professors and departments, and persons who strongly value academic freedom and scholarly pursuits, but who also support professional training, regional service and general education; (b) the power to change, or to make significant additions to the values allocated by campus governance generally was held not by these campus influentials alone but, historically, by such external authorities as the state government or a combination of external intervention and strategically placed, persistent internal leadership; (c) the central "power elite's" power was limited to decision choices within parameters set by departmental and professional autonomy, by historically rooted democratic norms and prevailing campus values, and by the monetary, regulatory, and policy powers of external groups; (d) although high position in governing committees and executive offices carried with it major influence, the faculty in general gained power by increasing its hold over the early stages of decision making— initiating concerns, gaining access to the agenda, controlling proposal study, formulation, and defense, and eventually making delegated decisions subject to review by formal authorities; (e) power accumulates as its source accumulates.[63]

Broad implications from this study indicate that those demonstrating support of more highly ranked values and norms are more likely than others to gain campus power and that those who control the stages of decision making in areas of academic affairs, personnel, finance, and capital development are more likely to wield power than others. The point made to acquire power is: (a) persuade or somehow get through the screening rituals and become an executive or faculty oligarch; (b) get in at the early stages of issue development —get the system of governance to deal with your concerns and knowledge; (c) bring pressure to bear; (d) if this fails to bring about change, autonomy as a teacher and researcher permits one to introduce change in your sphere of influence.[64]

As one searches the literature for theoretical formulations about power, the term becomes an all-enveloping concept with variables identified in number and in direct proportion to the number of authors reviewed. Bennis, in writing about the source of power, points out that its generation can be subtle (as through identification processes) or crude (in terms of rewards and punishment). There are four primary loci as sources of powers: (a) rewards and punishment, supplied by some exogenous agent; (b) self-control, generated through internalization of professional norms or standards of excellence (as designated by professional organizations or associations who designate standards for performance); (c) institutions of authority and contract as filtered through universalistic rules; and (d) group norms.[65]

Bennis defines power more specifically when he states that it is the perceived ability to control appropriate rewards and when it resides in an agent as leader leads to influence. He views leadership within a context that has three components—an agent as leader, manipulation of rewards—power, and induced behavior influence.[66]

Leininger conveys the sources of power from an anthropologic viewpoint when she designates the following methods: (a) interpersonal and persuasive techniques; (b) group alliances and coalitions; (c) a charismatic leadership style; (d) direct confrontation; (e) negotiation strategies; (f) revolution or overthrow of an existing individual or power group. Most nurse leaders tend to rely primarily on interpersonal and persuasive techniques, but hopefully, other methods will be tried in the future. Helping nurse administrators and leaders to become politicized and to select different power strategies according to the problem at hand is probably the greatest challenge.[67]

Ashley is eloquent in expressing her beliefs about power, generally, and specifically as it relates to nursing. She states that nursing has and always has had power. She views power as essentially social, derived from society's recognition of nursing as an essential service. "The problem lies in the ways in which nurses have used, misused, and abused (or failed to use it at all) and in the system in which nursing developed and is now practiced." [68] She goes on to point out that the desires of individuals and groups within the health care system have been of major significance in determining nursing's traditional role and power in the health field. Nursing's power struggle within the health care systems can be documented historically. This includes nursing's struggle (a) to attain a proper education for its practitioners though opposed, even today, by more powerful groups; (b) to throw off the burden of oppression imposed by those groups; (c) for the freedom to practice without numerous and professionally extraneous restraints and restrictions; (d) to convince others of the value and place of nursing in the health care system.[69]

Ashley points out that "The power of any group is relative, however, and must be understood within the context of the group's proximity to others who have power. There is no question but that many of nursing's conflicts and problems over power derive from the relationships established with other groups in the health field. And, certainly, the medical profession is one of the more politically powerful groups in both our society and our health care system." [69]

Schorr indicates that there is nothing wrong with power, rationally used and expressed. Without it there could be no change and nursing would be forever mired in a status quo.[70] Inherent in this statement is the implication that power can be bad. Power is neither good nor bad; how it is used determines its benefits or dangers. Bowman and Culpepper point out that nurses must be risk takers, identify goals, plan strategies, be accountable and responsible, and exercise authority. Only then can nurses determine the power they possess and/or the available source of potential power.[71] Power is defined as the ability to achieve goals that serve as the base for the acquisition and exercise of power and as a rallying point for members. The "effective exercise of power requires a theoretical or goal-oriented commitment, a thorough analysis of the situation at hand, and a willingness to take action to assume power at the appropriate time."[72] Power is a dynamic force charged by the interplay of human relationships; thus power does not exist in a vacuum and has an interpersonal dimension, as supported by Duncan and Tannenbaum et al.[73]

Gamson, in studying violence and political power, concludes that a group needs a bureaucratic structure to help become ready for action; it must have the willingness and the ability to fight, and the organization and discipline to focus its energy. Typically, strikes, bargaining, and propaganda were the primary means of influence, with violence viewed as the spice of protest but not the main substance. He found that every one who used violence successfully won new advantages and every recipient of violence was unsuccessful (excluded from the study were revolutionary groups aimed to displace the opposition). He goes on to conclude that it is disconcerting to discover that the meek do not inherit the earth or, at least, that portion of it presided over by the American political system. Groups choosing to fight their way into the political arena escape misfortune because they are prepared to withstand counterattack and to make it costly to those who would keep them out.[74]

Following on this extreme or negative orientation, McGregor's interpretation of power is that the usual implications of power as a controlling variable apply more appropriately to extreme forms of coercion. When he speaks of power he admits that the term influence would be more accurate. Some forms of power consist of influence brought to bear directly on people; others are indirectly applied by modifications in organizational environment through structure and managerial controls.[75] McGregor then looks at legitimate authority as one form of power basic to formal organizations of every kind. This form of power is manifested by day-to-day decision making, issuing orders, and establishing policies, procedures, and rules. Another source of power is evident in the direct control of extrinsic rewards (primarily money, but also vacations, travel, insurance, promotions) and punishments (demotion, suspension, discharge).[76] Any form of power rests on identification (when an individual genuinely identifies himself with a group, a leader, a cause) which serves as the basis for power. To maintain identification, movement toward relevant goals must be perceived. Finally, persuasive communication (means of giving information, expressing ideas and feelings and influencing others) is viewed as a form of power.[77]

These sources of power (legitimate authority, control of rewards and punishment, identification, and persuasive communication) are of value. Each also has limitations, with no one form inherently or generally more effective than any other. All forms of power are necessary causes of human behavior, but none is a sufficient cause. "The effectiveness of every form of power is limited—or *enhanced* . . . by the fact that all social influence is transactional in nature. There is virtually no such thing as unilateral influence because the human being (as well as the group or organization) is an open, organic system."[78]

Michael Korda adds still another dimension to the study and analysis of power by relating power to territoriality.

> To the person for whom work is the exercise of power, the place where it is done becomes the board on which power games are played, the central source from which power is derived. For at least eight hours a day the office provides one with all the risks, opportunities, dangers, triumphs, defeats, and demands of the larger world outside. It has its own landscape and nature features, which must be approached as the hunter approaches his environments; its own trails and paths and watering places, where the inhabitants can move and congregate in comparative freedom from the attention of predators; places where the natural color is good, and other places where danger can be scented, where the threat of the predator is in the air.[79]

He observes that offices are based upon a corner power system where the offices are larger and more desirable than in a central core. Distance from the corner offices designate the degree of power or powerlessness of the occupant. For example, the closer to the corner offices, the more power, while the closer one is to the physical center of the layout, the less powerful the person. "Power, therefore, tends to communicate itself from corner to corner in an X-shaped pattern, leaving certain areas as dead space, in power terms, even though they may contain large, comfortable rooms with outside windows."[79] Another territorial dimension, the floor level within an organization, is significant if in a large organization the center of power is on the lower two floors, with the more dispensible members of the organization on the upper stories of the building. "In ordinary power terms, however, a business in which the senior executives have retreated to a floor *below* their working staff is usually one in which the same seniors have also abdicated direct responsibility for day-to-day operations, allowing a separate and more active hierarchy to flourish above them unsupervised." [80] Color, too, has power significance and may be one of the simplest ways to establish control over space. Most people consider blue (reasonably dark, not sky blue or light blue) as the most powerful color. ". . . One can conclude that the most powerful combination of colors for an office would probably be white and dark blue, with perhaps accents of red here and there to inspire fear when necessary." [81]

Certain ways of placing furniture, too, can sometimes establish power rights. In many offices all desks in one department or one power area can be seen to face the same way, ie, toward the head of the department, in much the same fashion as Muslims in prayer would face Mecca. Offices can also be divided into direct confrontation areas (having desk and chairs) and social discussion areas (coffee table, sofa).[82]

One could question the purpose of or need for power. Rodgers has summarized the most distinguishing feature of power as relating to planned change.

> A primary feature of planned change is equal power distribution, that is, shared deliberations and goal setting. Both indoctrination (as practiced in many schools, prisons, and mental hospitals) and coercive change (thought control and brainwashing) are examples of an imbalanced power ratio, although indoctrinal change involves shared goal setting whereas coercive change does not. . . . In the world of medicine and health care delivery, power is generally sufficient to maintain things as they are.[83]

She views the reorganization or distribution of power as the role of the change agent. This change is accomplished by encouraging development of new sources of influence or making old power centers more responsive. Rodgers views fragmentation and competitiveness as related characteristics which have an impact on the change process. She sees the change agent as one whose task it is to turn intergroup competition into intergroup collaboration with the successful result in the direction of greater shared power.[83]

Duncan summarizes the major elements inherent in his discourse on power when he emphasizes the need for regular selective exercise of power. He views all exercises of power, which satisfy the *reasonable* needs of people, as the democratic exercise of power, such as approving good performance, rewarding sustained endeavor, and helping a colleague in difficulty. "These actions preserve and nurture the dignity and worth of the individual and contribute to his freedom." [84] Positive power exercised in the human society, which satisfies reasonable needs, is consistent with democratic leadership, whereas negative exercise of power (withholding of need satisfaction) is consistent with democratic principles when the denial is justified and serves the common good.[85]

Influence

The third term is influence. As with authority and power, considerable references can be gleaned from the literature. Influence is a highly significant term, directly applicable to the leadership process. Again, let's begin with Duncan, who defines influence as an interpersonal relationship devoid of power and authority and in which the behavior of one person affects that of another. Duncan believes that the influence relationship is a subtle one based upon some form of mutual trust and respect and built through social interaction. Whereas the exercise of authority and the exercise of power are fundamental to the generation of change, the influence relationship is needed to temper the effects of unlimited exercise of power and authority.[86]

In summarizing leadership as an exercise of influence, Stogdill believes that the influence concept shows that individuals differ in the impact their behaviors make on activities of the group. He says that influence implies a reciprocal relationship between leader and followers. This influence is not necessarily characterized by domination, control, or induction of compliance by the leader, but indicates that leadership exercises a determining effect on the behaviors of group members and on the activities of the group.[87]

Cartwright is another authority who has searched to determine the status of influence, leadership, and control. He identified three major aspects of the influence process: (a) the agent exerting influence, (b) the method of exerting influence, and (c) the agent subjected to influence. When an agent performs an act that causes some change in another agent, it can be said that the influencer has influenced the influencee and thus has power over the latter. Cartwright notes a problem in integrating the literature on the subject of influence when he points out that the agent (influencer) has at various times been an individual, a role, a position, a group, or a collection of people. There seems to be agreement among theorists, however, that the major base of influence is the possession, or control of valued resources, provided these can be used to facilitate or hinder another agent from attaining his goal.[88] When determining why a person attempts to exert influence, human motivation is considered in terms of gains and costs to be expected. When the influencer occupies a role, motivation is considered to be more complex because attempts to influence are guided, at least to some extent, by the expectations of others. Thus, the agent exerting influence is also influenced.

Cartwright continues with an exploration of the methods of influencing employed once the agent of influence and the motivation for exerting influence have been characterized. From the limited research directed to this aspect the following seven determinants may be operational. These are: (a) anticipation of the effectiveness of a given means; (b) evaluation of immediate costs; (c) assessment of delayed consequences; (d) general theory of human nature; (e) ethical evaluation of means; (f) position in social structure; (g) legal constraints.[89] "Influence or persuasion is essential if there is to be leadership, and the influence must be responsible or the leadership will be irresponsible." [90]

Tannenbaum et al state that the social process by which one individual attempts to influence one or more individuals is encountered in a large variety of interpersonal relationships, such as superior or subordinate, staff–line, consultant–client, salesman–customer, teacher–student, husband–wife, parent–child. This demands increased insight into numerous variables, such as personality, group, organization, and culture, with their interrelationship and interaction in a system of influence.[91]

Duncan views influence as the functional cornerstone of democratic leadership because the exercise of authority and power are only tolerable to free men when they can influence those who wield power and authority. In a democratic society, man can influence the decisions made and the way power is used to satisfy human needs. This involves affecting the behavior of those who have power and authority. Duncan believes that fundamental to influence is the element of mutuality, in which the leader is influenced by those led, and those led influence the leader. He points out that the greater the degree of mutual influence, the greater will be the power and authority exercised by the leader in effectively changing the behavior of the persons led. "An institutional position or office will carry with it some degree of authority and power but not influence." [92]

Dalton et al view influence from the standpoint of the formal organization. They believe that influence is a term with wider and broader connotations. Any successful direction or alteration in behavior represents influence, whether it is seen as legitimate or in violation of accepted values and quite apart from the means used to alter behavior. "In this sense, all authority is subsumed under the term influence, but there are certain types of influence, mainly coercive, which are not considered authority. . . ." [93]

Dalton et al view the initiation of change in an organization as essentially an episode in influence. To successfully initiate change, two prior conditions are needed (a) individuals involved are under stress and (b) the authority and power of the person initiating the changes must be viewed as a prestigious influencing figure. It is cautioned that the successful initiation of change, however, does not ensure that new behavior patterns will continue and persist. Non-organizational settings show the same link between prestige and influence in that individuals tend to behave and do the things suggested by authoritative prestigious sources.[94] Results of an organizational study of change, pointed out the most influential institutions in our society separate the individual whom they hope to influence from his regular social contacts and routines. The individual has been shown to demonstrate greater susceptibility to influence when he is separated from social contacts that support his current beliefs.[95]

For the individual to be influenced, the motivating force toward a particular change generally originates outside of the individual. He gradually accepts the influence when he deems the new ideas and prescribed actions are intrinsically rewarding in coping with internal and external stresses. Thus, when the change is internalized, the individual adopts the new behavior because he finds it relevant and valid in problem solving and consistent with his own views.[96]

To facilitate internalization of change as brought about through influence, the influencing person must introduce a framework of concepts. Dalton et al believe that this new framework of concepts may be restricted to a way of conceiving a limited set of phenomena. It could also be far-reaching in trying to explain the totality of a person's experience. "Implicit in the framework are relationships of acts to outcomes so that certain ends call for certain behavior. Finally, the influencing agent provides a language that not only communicates cognitive structure, but creates an 'associative net' by which the individual can relate the events in his own life to the new framework." [97]

The term "change" permeates most considerations of influence, authority, and power, with emphasis on the regular and selective use of authority and power tempered by the pervasive exercise of influence to create the most productive leadership for change.[98] A person can determine whether his influence is operating when he senses that the action of the other person seems completely voluntary and uncoerced.

Professional expertise and the exercise of authority, power, and influence presume that individuals have the professional expertise to discharge responsibility for their professional duties as demonstrated through educational credentials, licensing, and certification. The authority and power thus granted lie in professional matters, and the exercise of authority, power, and influence relationships will be constrained to the domain of the person's professional competence.[99]

To conclude, authority implies the right to make decisions affecting the behavior of others, whereas power is inherent in one's capacity to satisfy or not to satisfy human needs. Influence indicates a mutual and reciprocal relationship affecting the behavior of those to be influenced. In itself, influence is devoid of the characteristics of power and authority relationships. The three relationships involving authority, power, and influence are distinguishable in a conceptual, social, and professional sense, but are interdependent. Combined, they add a qualitative dimension to the study and exercise of leadership.[100] ". . . Influence in any form is a two-way process. The reactions of those influenced may not be directly or immediately observable to the influencer, but this does not mean they are absent." [101] The individual using influence may advise, suggest, discuss, persuade, or propagandize, but he does not exercise authority. He affects the behavior of another indirectly. But, influence can stem from the successful utilization of power with sensitivity, knowledge, and humanness to affect the behavior of others toward goal achievement.

ADMINISTRATION, MANAGEMENT, AND SUPERVISION

In addition to the concepts of authority, power, and influence, others are often used interchangeably with the term leadership, creating expectations that may not be appropriate and may be responsible for a lack of clarity or misinformation. Three such terms are administration, management, and supervision. In reviewing the literature on these terms, one is struck with the copious amount of available material. Terms are used freely, and interchangeably—often within the framework of the writings of a single author and frequently differing with the framework of other authors—resulting in confusion. In addition to the interchangeability of these three terms, they are frequently intermingled with the term leadership or even used interchangeably. The person who is the administrator, the manager, or the supervisor is also called the leader. Although leadership is certainly needed along with administration, management, and supervision, the latter terms have meaning within themselves. The success of the outcome of administration, management, and supervision may depend on the leadership process.

Although it is hoped that leadership behavior would be evident in conjunction with administration, management, and supervision, this may not be the case. Participation in administration, management, and supervision provides a framework wherein leadership may flourish. These terms are most likely associated with a formal organization and represent hierarchic positions. Concomitant task development is required to ensure that the goals of the formal organization are met. This does not mean that leadership may not be evident within the formal organization or in any aspect of these positions in the hierarchic structure. Persons can function within these positions by virtue of the authority inherent in each without demonstrating leadership behavior, providing they have the necessary expertise to implement policy and to see that tasks are completed as predicted and expected.

Leadership is free standing and not limited to the formal organization. The leadership behavior so needed and prized cannot be structured for selected settings but is inherent in the individual.

Administration, management, and supervision are terms that belong in formal organizations. These terms have distinct similarities and differences as well as demonstrated common features. They are frequently associated with authority, power, and influence.

Administration is viewed as the broadest, most encompassing term, followed by management which although a more specific term, is considered a dimension of administration in the formal organization. Supervision is the narrowest, most self-limiting of the terms, being classified under administration as well as management.

To validate the relationship between these three terms as viewed by the authors, these terms, along with the term leadership, were given to groups of graduate (N-104) and undergraduate (N-21) students in nursing. The students were asked to define and order the four terms. The responses indicated that the majority felt that leadership was the most encompassing term followed by administration. Management was ordered third by a very narrow margin, being contrasted closely with supervision. Most of the students regarded supervision as a third or fourth priority, ie, 20 placed it third and 21 fourth. These results support the authors' contentions. There was no doubt that leadership was the broadest most permeating concept.

Discrimination between administration and management was less widespread. This same pattern prevailed for ordering management and supervision (see Appendix).

The following presentation contains simple definitions of these terms and presents some of the prevailing notions based on a survey of the literature. The presentation is in no way intended to cover the topic, but is basic to contrast the difference between these terms and leadership so as to help the reader focus more precisely on the latter term without the strain of term interchange.

Administration

Administration, as the broadest of these hierarchic terms, means direction and conduction of persons collectively involved with the execution of policy and/or laws. Shanks and Kennedy define administration as "that organization through which persons in a given social setting achieve a desired and defined goal." [102] These authors define nursing service administration as an "organization through which nurses in a hospital or another type of health agency were able to provide the best possible nursing care for patients in the hospital or under the jurisdiction of another type of health agency." [102] An administrative process viewed as a scientific process has been delineated, consisting of the components thinking, planning, communicating, gaining group acceptance, organizing, delegating, guiding and evaluating to plan to meet client care needs, directing the care, arranging and controlling the setting, and facilitating the accomplishment of care.[103] It is stated that in relation to the performance of an administrative function, thinking is the essence, the core from which action originates.[104] Other authors have indicated that the administrative process includes decision making, programming, communicating, controlling, and reappraising. Rotkovitch points out that the necessary administrative skills include leading, directing, motivating, organizing, being fiscally responsible, evaluating, and recommending. The administrator has the difficult task of coordinating and allocating, in an equitable fashion, all available human and material resources to achieve the best care possible.[105] Additional components of the administrative process include tasks of an executive nature—organizing, policy making, staffing, organizational planning and budget, delegating, direct contact with nursing personnel, and/or coordinating and evaluating nursing service.[106]

From the point of view of educational administration, Griffiths indicates that administration has some aspects of an art. Inquiry in administration should be objective, reliable, contain operational definitions, have a coherent or systematic structure, and demonstrate comprehensiveness. Likewise, a theory of administration should provide guides to action, to the collection of facts, and to new knowledge.[107]

The statements of assumptions underlying a theory of administration as decision making, proposed by Griffiths, are the following:

1. Administration is a generalized type of behavior to be found in all human organizations.
2. Administration is the process of directing and controlling life in a social organization.
3. The specific function of administration is to develop and regulate the decision-making process in the most effective manner possible.
4. The administration works with groups or with individuals with a group referent, not with individuals as such.

Related concepts include not only decision making, but organization, perception, communication, power, and authority.[108]

Gallagher includes a discourse on educational administration in nursing, specifically geared to the administration of a baccalaureate program in a college or university. Areas of focus for educational administration include the curriculum, student personnel services, the faculty, the budget, interrelationships and collaboration, research and program evaluation.[109] Still others include decision making, communicating, planning, controlling, influencing, coordinating, and evaluating as components of the administrative process. Some of these authors combine components of the leadership process with the administrative process.

It seems evident that there is an administrative process. Various authors seem to consistently designate decision making, policy making, directing and controlling, budgeting, delegating, conducting, organizing, and evaluating, as process components. The administrative process flourishes in the hierarchic formal organization.

It may be useful to explore the dimensions of hierarchy and outline some of the theoretical formulations in existence at the present time. It has been stated that hierarchy exists in nearly all organizations, with its vertical levels of authority, its division of labor, and the connotation of a status ranging from highest to lowest.[110] But this is a narrow view of hierarchy and limited to formal organizations. Hierarchy is significant in the whole of nature. Pattee, in his presentation on hierarchy theory, points out that it is a "central lesson of biological evolution that increasing complexity of organization is always accompanied by new levels of hierarchical controls. The loss of these controls at any level is usually malignant for the organization under that level. . . . Loss of hierarchical controls often results in sudden and catastrophic failure." [111] He continues, "at each level we must learn to abstract what is most significant, for what is true in detail at a lower level does not usually give us a clear picture of the upper level." [112] Simon delineates four intertwined hierarchic sequences to explain most of the complex systems in nature. These are: (a) the hierarchy in observable chemical substances comprised of sets of molecules, which, in turn, are comprised of atoms, nuclei, and electrons, and, finally, within the nuclei are elementary particles; (b) the hierarchy which runs from living organisms to tissues and organs, to cells, to macromolecules, to organic compounds; (c) the hierarchy which leads from the statistics of inheritance to genes and chromosomes, to DNA, and others; (d) the hierarchy, not yet firmly connected with the others, which lead to human beings, to cognitive programs in the central nervous system, to elementary information processes where the functions with the tissues and organs of neurobiology largely remain to be discovered. Inherent in this fourth sequence are programs and elementary information processes occurring increasingly in the artificial, complex systems of digital computers.[113]

All large systems have hierarchic organization. Most interactions in nature have been found to occur between systems of all kinds and to decrease in strength with distance. Any given particle or element interacts most strongly with others nearby, resulting in a system that behaves as a collection of localized subsystems or forming a somewhat uniform "tissue" or cohesive element of equally strong interactions.[114] "Hierarchy is associated with a very fundamental form of parsimony of interactions." [115] The significance of hierarchic organization is crucial to the synthesis and survival of large complex systems.

Simon indicates that the functional efficacy of the higher level hierarchic structures and their stability, can be made relatively independent of the detail of their microscopic components. The several components on any given level of the hierarchy can preserve a measure of independence, adapting to their special aspects of the environment without destroying their usefulness to the total system.[116]

Grobstein observes that the living world may be viewed as populations in higher sets called *communities* and that persons within these communities may be viewed as collections or sets of units. An understanding and appreciation of the levels of order and of hierarchic systems is essential to an understanding of life itself. "In its simplest sense hierarchic order refers to a complex of successively more encompassing sets. In hierarchies a given set must be described not only for itself but in terms both of what is within *it* and what it is *within*." [117]

A set is considered a level of order in the hierarchic system. This set is thought to consist of identifiable components which comprise a level or order in which the components are in a determinate association, making up the sum of the relationships of the components. Thus a set is a level of order having unitary properties, at that particular level, stemming from particular relationships among and properties of its components.[118] A sand pile whose grains of sand contribute to its weight, color, and shape is given as an example. The sand grains themselves are indistinguishable as to their properties, whether they are within the pile or out of it. In living systems, components almost always have different properties, depending upon the context of the system within which they operate. This functional adaptability of living units is one of their prime characteristics; they do not merely aggregate, they form a collective unit. Yet such collectives frequently are reversible, they form or disband depending upon circumstances or preference.[119]

Grobstein concludes by saying hierarchic order is characteristic of living systems, and that hierarchic organizations in biologic systems display an array of delicately and intricately interlocked orders that steadily increase in level and complexity.[120] Pattee takes this concept a point further by recognizing structural hierarchies in both living and nonliving matter. However, he points out that the distinguishing characteristic of life is the *control* hierarchy. This implies a narrower partial ordering that indicates the upper level has active authority over elements of the lower levels.[121] Pattee further elaborated additional constraints imposed by some authority over individuals living in a group. This constraining authority is not just one ordinary individual of the group to whom a title is given such as admiral or president. When the origin of this authority was traced, it was found that the constraints are more accurately called group constraints executed by an individual holding an office established by a collective hierarchic organization.[122] Control is another dimension that must be considered. Pattee indicates that control implies constraint or regulation of a total system, whereas function often applies to a specific process that is only a small part of the whole organism.[123] ". . . Hierarchical controls arise from a degree of internal constraint that forces the elements into a collective, simplified behavior independent of selected details of the dynamic behavior of its elements." [124] He indicates that hierarchic control operates between levels and is a problem of the nature of the interface between levels, characterized by the principles of classification of detail (microscopic degrees of freedom, eg, molecule), optimum constraint (not too numerous or tight or too scarce or loose) and statistical closure (the variety of alternative descriptions and functions unlimited by the fixed set of structural elements comprising the constraints of the organization).[125] Lemin supports this connotation when she states that control is an inevitable correlate of organization, necessary to help circumscribe idiosyncrasies of behavior, help members conform, and give members the requirements to meet objectives of the organization.[126]

Pattee concludes that in determining the direction for the development and application of hierarchy theory there is an apparent paradox. There can never be a closed system of hierarchies, like a dynamic theory in physics, because managing a system implies adding at least one hierarchic level to oversee the system, ie, the management level. "Hierarchy theory must be more like theories of language or programming that give us useful rules or methods for the most effective design and control of open-ended systems that can continually grow and evolve new levels." [127] This involves the most common and most concrete concept associated with hierarchic organization—the concept of discrete interacting levels. Simon postulates that levels originate in two ways: structure and description. He feels that the speed of evolution of complex systems will favor those with stable intermediate structural levels and complex systems are incomprehensible unless they are simplified by using alternative levels of description, such as the computer which needs several levels of description for effective programming.[128]

In regard to the applicability of these concepts to the terms administration, management, and supervision, which are under discussion, predicting and controlling the behavior of a system are important concepts. When coupled with levels of structure and description, it follows that any notion of administration, management, and supervision, or any form of control for that matter, must operate between two hierarchic levels. "This is true for any informational constraints where structural alternatives on one level are subordinated by a higher level descriptive process. This is the case in all forms of a decision making, classification, recognition, or measurement process." [129]

The reason the two levels of structure and description are needed for any prediction and control process is that (a) in order to predict how a system will behave, it must be assumed it can only behave one way without the possibility of some alternative behavior; and (b) to control a system it must be assumed that alternative behaviors are possible.[129] Administration then is considered to be an encompassing term inherent in any formal organization with a hierarchic structure. Authority is inherent in the structure, varying in degree and power, ie, authority and power are maximal at the highest hierarchic level and least at the lowest hierarchic level. Administration is a process needed to ensure the viability of formal organization; it comprises the active means to fulfill the purposes of a formal organization. Decision making, controlling, delegating, planning, coordinating, and evaluating behaviors are required of person(s) designated to administrate. It means providing the policies and methods needed to fulfill objectives as well as for marshaling the human and physical resources needed for policy making, executive action, and control. The placement of authority and the use of power depend on the number of levels inherent in the organization, the extent to which authority and power are delegated in conjunction with responsibility, the effectiveness of decision making, and the acceptability of decisions made to the large numbers of persons at the lowest hierarchic level who put those decisions into operation. Another important dimension is the direction of communication—from top to bottom only, bottom to top only, top to bottom and bottom to top continuously. A break in communication at any place from top to bottom or bottom to top creates problems, if not disaster for the formal organization.

Management

Management is viewed as a component within the broad framework of administration. Management is less encompassing and is more closely linked to specific levels in the hierarchic structure of the organization. Management is defined as the conduct or direction of anything, including wielding, controlling, dealing, carrying on and handling. Gill feels that management is conceptual and cannot be expressed as a concise concept. Rather, it is a growing, loosely formed association of concepts, gaining in unity and acceptance with time.[130] Others believe management means organizing, guiding, controlling, activating, and evaluating human and physical resources into functional units that accomplish a task. It means control of the process of executing given policy and is clearly distinguished from the formulation and determination of policy and the activities involved and abilities required, which are seen as administration.[131]

Tannenbaum synthesizes the efforts of many authors when he designates organization and delegation as strategic components of the management process. To organize means to relate to units or parts, each having its proper or special task to perform, and an arrangement involving an interdependence or relationship between the units or parts. Inherent in this is the determination of the degree and type of specialization to be put into operation within the formal organization, and a determination of the relationships needed among specialized units.[132] To delegate means to invest a person with formal authority to act for another. This investiture is always within specified and orderly defined limits of authority. To delegate formal authority to subordinates carries responsibility for this exercise to a superior who, in turn, delegated it to him. This delegation of authority to subordinates may be described as authority to prescribe (indicate how designated activities shall be performed) and enforce (see that activities are performed).[133] Once management has determined the type and intensity of specialization to be effectuated (within the formal organization) and the relationships that are to exist among specialized units, it follows that mechanisms of direction come into play. Formal authority is used in this way to guide subordinates. It involves devising the purposes of action and the methods or procedures to be followed in achieving them.[134] A component of direction is control, which involves the use of formal authority to ensure, to the extent possible, that the purposes of action are attained by the methods and procedures devised.

According to Alexander, management is viewed as a process for maintaining the internal environment to achieve organized effort to accomplish group objectives.[135] The management process includes planning, organizing, controlling, and communicating.[136] The heart of management involves taking effective action, having a clear conception of goals, having a plan of action, being prepared to take action, and being able to communicate goals, operational plans, strategies, organizational structure, and the results of action.[137]

Thus, management is the use of delegated authority, within the formal organization, to organize, direct, or control responsible subordinates (indirectly, this includes the groups or complexes which they may head), so that all service contributions are coordinated to attain a goal. Tannenbaum et al state that a person is a manager and manages only if he has and uses formal authority to organize, direct, or control responsible subordinates. He is a nonmanager unless he conforms to these specifications.[138] Tannenbaum et al state further that the services of manager, as stated above, are necessary only to coordinate the specialized service contributions of units he heads to achieve the enterprise purpose and for no other reason.[139] Schurr makes a point of distinguishing between scientific management and the philosophy or art of management. She ascribes policy making, planning, organization, decision making, control, and problem solving to scientific management, while social skills, behavioral aspects, working with groups, environmental factors, human relationships indicate the philosophy and art of management, with leadership being an integral part.[140]

Thus, in a sense, management is restricted in that it involves mechanisms required to accomplish a task through subordinates, as delegated by a higher authority. Management is inherent in the larger framework of administration. But, its purpose is always in the direction of attaining the purposes of the formal organization rather than designating these purposes. Management is responsible to a higher authority and, in this sense, it is subordinate to administration.

Supervision

Supervision is the narrowest of the terms and may be described as a unit within the aspect of management in the formal organization. The act of supervision is closest to the hierarchic level where specific activities are operationalized, having been appropriately delegated from other hierarchic levels. It is indispensable and needed to ensure the detailed performance of work or service.

Supervision means to oversee for regulation, to inspect, to peruse. It is viewed as a dynamic process in which the supervising person encourages or participates in the development of subordinates.[141]

Bowers and Seashore make a point of differentiation for supervision. They state that the supervisory role is one of greater emphasis on planning and performing specialized skill tasks. This includes behavior that delegates authority, provides generalized instruction, allows individuals to perform in their own way at their own pace, supports personal relationships, and fosters group cohesiveness and pride.[142] Additional elements delineated for supervision are intercommunication and interpretation, encouragement, improvement, and participation. McGregor noted a shift in the supervisory role from one of direction, surveillance, and control to one of providing technical help, support, and instruction.[143]

Thus, supervision is viewed as that component of administration closest to persons who perform the services and do the work needed to meet formal organizational objectives. The processes inherent in supervision include planning, communication, direction, instruction, technical assistance, support, and evaluation. The scope of impact for supervision is narrower, in a sense, than management but more directly involved with the persons responsible for tasks. Supervision of subordinates at the lowest level of the hierarchy involves the final track for delegation. The number of persons involved in supervision is larger than the number in management, which, in turn, is larger than the number needed for administration.

Thus, administration, management, and supervision are terms that indicate survival for a formal organization that has a precise purpose to fulfill. They are terms associated with the formal organization designed in levels—hierarchic in structure. Most formal authority, as power, is vested in higher levels of the hierarchy. Formal authority and power can be delegated to and shared with all levels of the hierarchy. Control is a dimension readily seen in formal organization when administration, management, and supervision are reviewed.

The three terms discussed have value and meaning in their own right and are not interchangeable with the term leadership. Although a combination of leadership and administration, management, and supervision may be desirable and needed, administration, management, and supervision alone do not imply this. Leadership must be viewed as a separate entity. Further, an administrator is not automatically a leader and a leader is not automatically an administrator. This holds true for managers and supervisors.

The following observations were gleaned from various reports about administration, management, and supervision.

1. Administration, management, and supervision are associated with formal organization.
2. Hierarchic theory has developed and contributes in part to an explanation of hierarchy in nature.
3. The term control is far more prevalent in the literature concerned with administration, management, and supervision than it is found with leadership.
4. A control process is an integral part of administration, management, and supervision.

5. The administration process, management process, and supervision process have been determined.
6. The activities associated with administration, supervision, and management range from policy determination to the overseeing of and carrying out of policy as denoted by management and delegating the actual carrying out of policy at the employee level.
7. Administration is the broadest term, management is intermediate, and supervision is related to function at the policy implementation level—the level at which purposes of a formal organization are achieved—and is the narrowest term.
8. Some components in the processes of administration, management, and supervision are common to each and some may be common to the leadership process.
9. How the total processes of administration, management, and supervision within the formal organization are viewed determines and limits each term.

In this chapter, the authors discussed the concepts and theories related to leadership. Nursing leadership per se is explored in Chapter 3.

References

1. Webster's New World Dictionary of the American Language. New York, World Publishing Co, 1960, p. 99.
2. *Idem:* p 99.
3. *Idem:* p 749.
4. Webster's New Twentieth Century Dictionary of the English Language, unabridged. New York, Standard Reference Works Publishing Co, 1956.
5. Duncan J: The curriculum director in curriculum change. Educ Forum 38:51, Nov, 1973.
6. *Idem:* p 52.
7. *Idem:* p 53.
8. *Idem:* pp 53-54.
9. Merton R: The social nature of leadership. Am J Nurs 69:2615, 1969.
10. Bennis W: Leadership theory and administrative behavior. Admin Sci Q 4:289, 1959.
11. Dalton G, Barnes L, Zaleznik A: The Distribution of Authority in Formal Organization. Cambridge, MIT Press, 1968, pp 37-38.
12. *Idem:* p 38.

13. *Idem:* pp 38-39.
14. *Idem:* p 39.
15. *Idem:* p 45.
16. Barnard C: The Functions of the Executive. Cambridge, Harvard University Press, 1964, p 173.
17. Dalton G, Barnes L, Zaleznik A: The Distribution of Authority in Formal Organization. Cambridge, MIT Press, 1968, p 150.
18. Thompson V: Modern Organization. New York, Alfred Knopf, 1961, p 6.
19. Kalisch B: Of half gods and mortals: aesculapian authority. Nurs Outlook 23:23, Jan 1975.
20. Tannenbaum R, Weschler I, Massarik F: Leadership and Organization. New York, McGraw-Hill Book Co, 1961, p 271.
21. *Idem:* pp 272-273.
22. *Idem:* p 274.
23. Clark B: Faculty organization and authority, Academic Governance. Edited by JV Baldridge, Berkeley, Calif, McCutchan Publishers, 1971, p 237.
24. *Idem:* p 238.
25. *Idem:* p 242.
26. *Idem:* pp 243-45.
27. *Idem:* pp 246-47.
28. *Idem:* p 247.
29. *Idem:* p 249.
30. Blau P: The Organization of Academic Work. New York, John Wiley and Sons, 1973, p 158.
31. *Idem:* p 161.
32. *Idem:* p 186.
33. *Idem:* p 188.
34. Dalton G, Barnes L, Zaleznik A: The Distribution of Authority in Formal Organization. Cambridge, MIT Press, 1968, p 148.
35. Duncan J: The curriculum director in curriculum change. Educ Forum 38:57, Nov, 1973.
36. *Idem:* p 57.
37. *Idem:* p 54.
38. Dalton G, Barnes L, Zaleznik A: The Distribution of Authority in Formal Organization. Cambridge, MIT Press, 1968, p 40.
39. *Idem:* p 41.
40. *Idem:* pp 42-43 (footnote).
41. *Idem:* p 42.
42. *Idem:* p 43.
43. *Idem:* p 47.
44. *Idem:* p 49.
45. *Idem:* p 50.
46. *Idem:* p 147.
47. Griffiths D: Administrative Theory. New York, Appleton-Century-Crofts, 1959, pp 86-87.

48. Tannenbaum R, Weschler I, Massarik F: Leadership and Organization. New York, McGraw-Hill Book Co, 1961, p 26.
49. Stogdill R: Handbook of Leadership. New York, Free Press, 1974, p 293.
50. *Idem:* p 292-293.
51. Mott P: Power, authority, and influence, The Structure of Community Power. Edited by M Aiken, P Mott. New York, Random House, 1970, p 10.
52. *Idem:* p 11.
53. *Idem:* p 11.
54. *Idem:* pp 14-15.
55. *Idem:* p 15.
56. Hawley W, Wirt F: The Search for Community Power. Englewood Cliffs, NJ, Prentice-Hall, 1968, p 2.
57. Blau P: On the Nature of Organizations. New York, John Wiley and Sons, 1974, pp 19-20.
58. Etzioni A: Organizational control structure. Handbook of Organizations. Edited by J. March. Chicago, Rand McNally, p 650.
59. *Idem:* p 651.
60. *Idem:* p 655.
61. *Idem:* p 660.
62. Lindquist J, Blackburn R: Middlegrove: the locus of campus power at a state university. AAUP Bull 60:367-68, 1974.
63. *Idem:* pp 376-377.
64. *Idem:* p 378.
65. Bennis W: Leadership theory and administrative behavior. Admin Sci Q 4:290, 1959.
66. *Idem:* p 296.
67. Leininger M: The leadership crisis in nursing: a critical problem and challenge. J Nurs Admin, 40:32, 1974.
68. Ashley JA: This I believe about power in nursing. Nurs Outlook 21:638, 1973.
69. *Idem:* p 638.
70. Schorr T: Nurse power. Am J Nurs 74:1047, 1974
71. Bowman R, Culpepper R: Power: Rx for change. Am J Nurs 74:1053, 1974.
72. *Idem:* p 1054.
73. *Idem:* p 1056.
74. Gamson W: Violence and political power: the meek don't make it. Psychol Today 80:39-41, July 1974.
75. McGregor D: The Professional Manager. New York, McGraw-Hill Book Co, 1967, p 137.
76. *Idem:* pp 138-142.
77. *Idem:* pp 145-150.
78. *Idem:* pp 154-155.
79. Korda M: Office power—you are where you sit. New York 8:36, January 13, 1975.

80. *Idem:* pp 39-40.
81. *Idem:* p 43.
82. *Idem:* p 44.
83. Rodgers J: Theoretical considerations involved in the process of change. Nurs Forum 12:171-172, 1973.
84. Duncan J: The curriculum director in curriculum change. Educ Forum 38:60, Nov, 1973.
85. *Idem:* p 61.
86. *Idem:* pp 55-56.
87. Stogdill R: Handbook of Leadership. New York, Free Press, 1974, p 10.
88. Cartwright D: Influence, leadership, control, Handbook of Organizations. Edited by J. March. Chicago, Rand-McNally, 1965, p 11.
89. *Idem:* p 21.
90. Lansing K: Weaknesses in teacher education. Educ Forum 38:32, November 1973.
91. Tannenbaum R, Weschler I, Massarik F: Leadership and Organization. New York, McGraw-Hill Book Co, 1961, p 2.
92. Duncan J: The curriculum director in curriculum change. Educ Forum 38:62, Nov, 1973.
93. Dalton G, Barnes L, Zaleznik A: The Distribution of Authority in Formal Organization. Cambridge, MIT Press, 1968, p 37.
94. *Idem:* p 115.
95. *Idem:* p 124.
96. *Idem:* p 139.
97. *Idem:* p 140.
98. Duncan J: The curriculum director in curriculum change. Educ Forum 38:63, Nov, 1973.
99. *Idem:* p 65.
100. *Idem:* p 57.
101. McGregor D: The Professional Manager. New York, McGraw-Hill Book Co, 1967, p 15.
102. Shanks M, Kennedy D: The Theory and Practice of Nursing Service Administration. New York, McGraw-Hill Book Co, 1965, p 3.
103. *Idem:* pp 4, 109.
104. *Idem:* p 111.
105. Rotkovitch R: The director of nursing and the hat of administration. J NY State Nurse Assoc 4:40-43, Nov 1973.
106. Young L: Room at the top . . . a place for nurse administrators. J Nurs Admin 00:82, Nov-Dec, 1972.
107. Griffiths D: Administrative Theory. New York, Appleton-Century-Crofts, 1959, p 45.
108. *Idem:* pp 71-74, 91.
109. Gallagher A: Educational Administration in Nursing. New York, Macmillan Co, 1965, pp xiii-xiv.
110. Looking into nursing leadership. In Leadership in Nursing Monograph. Washington, Leadership Resources Inc, 1966, p 14.

111. Hierarchy Theory: The Challenge of Complex Systems. Edited by H. Pattee. New York, George Braziller, 1973, p xi.
112. *Idem:* p xii.
113. *Idem:* pp 5-6.
114. *Idem:* p 9.
115. *Idem:* p 15.
116. *Idem:* pp 23-24.
117. *Idem:* p 31.
118. *Idem:* pp 31-32.
119. *Idem:* p 33.
120. *Idem:* pp 46-47.
121. *Idem:* pp 75-76.
122. *Idem:* p 78.
123. *Idem:* p 81.
124. *Idem:* p 93.
125. *Idem:* p 105.
126. Lemin B: Organizations and their processes. Nurs Times 69:93, June 14, 1973.
127. Pattee H: Unsolved problems and potential applications of hierarchy theory. In Hierarchy Theory: The Challenge of Complex Systems. Edited by H. Pattee. New York, George Braziller, 1973, p 132.
128. *Idem:* pp 132-133.
129. *Idem:* p 142.
130. Gill W: Key concepts in management in nursing. Superv Nurse: 20:21, 1971.
131. Tannenbaum R, Weschler I, Massarik F: Leadership and Organization. New York, McGraw-Hill Book Co, 1961, p 252.
132. Idem: pp 254-255.
133. *Idem:* p 257.
134. *Idem:* p 258.
135. Alexander E: Nursing Administration in the Hospital Health Care System. St. Louis, CV Mosby Co, 1972, p 90.
136. *Idem:* p 93.
137. *Idem:* p 91.
138. Tannenbaum R, Weschler I, Massarik F: Leadership and Organization. New York, McGraw-Hill Book Co, 1961, p 263.
139. *Idem:* p 264.
140. Schurr M: A comparative study of leadership in industry and the nursing profession, Part I. Int Nurs Rev 16:17, 1969.
141. Perrodin C: Supervision of Nursing Service Personnel. New York, Macmillan Co, 1954, p 10.
142. Bowers DG, Seashore SE: Predicting organizational effectiveness with a four-factor theory leadership. Leadership. Edited by CA Gibbs. Baltimore, Penguin Books, 1969, p 363.
143. McGregor D: The Professional Manager. New York, McGraw-Hill Book Co, 1967, p 91.

CHAPTER 3
Nursing Leadership

There is no shortage of materials, thoughts, or ideas about leadership since it is a topic that has concerned men and women throughout the ages. It has been a fascination to want to predict who will become a leader, to discover what a leader does, to find out what a leader is, and what makes the differences. Why are some people designated as leaders while others are not? There are a number of literature surveys available related to leadership. The most notable is that of Ralph Stogdill.[1] No attempt will be made to duplicate the surveys. But, the extensive literature on leadership limits our ability to use what is available.

As the research on leadership and leadership skills comes into the foreground, more and more frequently leadership is being viewed as a very complex situation involving leaders, followers, situations, and all variables that have an impact on them. This includes needs of the leader and followers, internal pressures, external pressures, interaction among these variables, and the environment in which they exist. Considerable work has been done related to varying styles of leadership, including the finding that one leadership style may be useful at one time but not at another. One individual may need to use different leadership styles to achieve designated goals. In short, the present state of knowledge concerning leadership may stimulate the realization that a lot, yet very little, is known about leadership per se.

This chapter focuses on aspects of leadership and leadership theory, selectively chosen, that explain and foster the development of leadership in nursing. The elements and theories or theoretical formulations included have been carefully selected. Components of leadership, which is viewed as a process, will be designated. How these components influence the action of leadership, how leadership differs from authority, and the effect of the role of authority, power, and influence on nursing leadership will also be discussed.

In a formal organization there are many positions in which leadership may or may not be needed. Only when an individual uses the leadership process can it be determined whether or not that individual exhibited leadership behavior, regardless of the situation involved. This does not contradict the idea that the situation is an important variable of leadership. We will focus our attention on the nurse who demonstrates the leadership process in any nursing situation.

Certain assumptions should be considered in any discussion of leadership in nursing.

1. Nursing is viewed as an interpersonal process. It involves an encounter between nurse and client, with the expressed purpose of fostering maximum well-being on the part of the client whether that client is an individual, a family, or groups of individuals or families. Where recovery from illness is impossible, the nurse strives to add a dimension of comfort, compassion, and care until life ends.
2. Leaders in nursing can be deliberately prepared. No particular combination or collection of traits and personality characteristics have been identified for leaders, which, in fact, are not found in the general population of persons who are not leaders. There seems to be a strong indication that the leadership process can be learned; therefore, the discourse presented on nursing leadership is expected to serve as a framework for the development of nursing leaders.
3. A shortage of nursing leadership behavior exists at the present time. Nurses have been known to ponder the few valiant leaders

who made an impact on nursing in the past and are concerned that these types of individuals are not heard of today. At least part of the reason for this lack can be attributed to the increased complexity of nursing today, so that few individuals have the opportunity to make a direct impact. Nursing leadership at the present time is much more diffuse than in earlier eras. Today, many individuals are indeed demonstrating leadership behavior, as envisioned by the writers, but may not receive the national recognition afforded persons such as Isabel Hampton Robb, Florence Nightingale, or Isabel Stewart.

LEADERSHIP THEORETICAL FORMULATIONS

From a review of the contributions of many scholars in the field of leadership, it would seem that the theoretical formulations proposed by Tannenbaum, Weschler, and Massarik have the greatest utility in nursing and will serve as a pivot point. In addition, theoretical formulations of other authors have been selected in an attempt to (a) distinguish and develop elements of the leadership process; (b) determine dimensions that affect leadership, such as power, influence, coercion, authority, and (c) demonstrate the distinction between leadership, administration, management, and supervision, with leadership permeating all areas. Administration, management, and supervision are limited to formal organizations and consist of certain predetermined lines of authority and techniques available for use by individuals—who may or may not demonstrate leadership behavior.

Inherent in leadership is the concept of change. To proceed from goal setting to goal achievement constitutes a change and the leader plays a large part in energizing and promoting this change in a positive, useful, and socially acceptable direction. The weight, direction, and extent of change will be determined by the complexity of the situation, the number of variables, the number of people involved, and the acceptability of determined goals. The composition and consensus of the group will influence goal achievement as well as the rate and amount of change within individuals and the environment needed to achieve the required goal.

Gibbs comments that at this time in the history of mankind no strong theory of leadership exists, in the sense that explanations and predictions may be made which would apply widely to many people in many groups and many places. Until, and unless, research findings are incorporated in a theory of leadership, which at the same time fits and runs beyond it, findings will lack value. Ideas and facts must be incorporated into practice to have meaning. "Theory it is which casts up hypotheses for further research and propositions in trial application in situations of greater complexity and wider scope. The basic aim of science is theory, that is to say to find general explanations of natural events." [2]

Thus, the theoretical considerations selected are drawn from the general frame of reference of numerous authors, but mainly from Tannenbaum, Weschler, and Massarik, who considered the leader and his psychologic attributes, the follower, the group, the situation, interpersonal relationships, and communication. These authors developed a useful frame of reference for leadership that may be applied to nursing. They define leadership as *"interpersonal influence, exercised in situation and directed, through the communication process, toward the attainment of a specified goal or goals."* [3] Leadership is viewed as attempts on the part of the leader to affect the behavior of a follower or followers in a given situation. In other words, the influencer influences the behavior of the influencee in a situation.

Interpersonal influence is considered the essence of leadership, with the leader attempting to affect the behavior of followers through communication. A person who attempts to influence others, successfully or unsuccessfully, is viewed as a leader. The assessment of leadership effectiveness is considered a separate matter.

Power has a potential for influence, but an individual, because of personal values, an apparent lack of need or misjudgment, may not use all of the power available to him. "A leadership act reflects that portion of the power available to an individual which he chooses to employ at the time." Not only are external sources of power available to a leader but so is power derived from inner resources, such as understanding and flexibility.[4]

Situation is defined as those aspects of the objective context (physical phenomenon, other individuals, the organization, the broader culture with its social norms, role prescriptions and goals —personal, group, and organizational) which, at any particular time, have an attitudinal or behavioral impact on individuals in the influence relationship. It is recognized that the situaton of the leader and that of the follower may differ in many respects.[5]

Leadership, in this framework, concerns only the interpersonal influence that can be exercised through communication processes. Physical manipulation and coercion, in their pure forms, are not included. Threats or other coercive devices imparted by communication only are considered. Communication is the sole process through which a leader, as such, can function. The goal of the communicator is to transmit a message (meanings or ideas) from himself to a communicatee so that it is received as intended without distortion.[6]

The leader uses communication not only to change attitudes but as a medium through which he tries to affect the followers' attitudes so that the follower will be ready to or will move in the direction of a specified goal. To be effective a leader needs to select communication behaviors that are likely to have an impact on the follower's personality in such a way that attitudes are changed and behavior is goal directed.[7]

The goals toward which the leader exerts his influence may be categorized as organizational, group, and personal (leader and follower). For organizational goals, which are those of the organization and may have little or no direct motivational importance, the leader may use inducements relevant to the need systems of the followers. In contrast, group goals are those that evolve through interaction of group members and reflect what the group decides. The leader who emerges is one who influences members through his sensitivity toward the objectives and his skill in effecting their fulfillment.

The personal goals of the follower are met when the leader uses his influence to establish an atmosphere of warmth, security, and acceptance, and through interpersonal techniques aids another to reach ends that could not possibly be reached alone. The leader's personal goals, whether on a conscious or unconscious level, may be met primarily through his influence. These goals may coexist with organizational or group goals.[6]

Effectiveness in leadership, as seen by Tannenbaum, Weschler, and Massarik, is a function of interrelationships between the personality characteristics of the leader and those of the follower as well as the characteristics of the situation within the field of each individual.

> . . . the *situation* has a different impact on both the leader and the follower as they interact. The *personality of the follower* (as it manifests itself in a given situation) becomes the key variable with which the leader must deal. The needs, attitudes, values, and feelings of the follower determine the kinds of stimuli the leader must use to make the follower respond. The *personality of the leader* (also becomes manifest in a situation) influences his range of perception of the followers and situation, his judgment of what is relevant among these perceptions, and therefore his sensitivity to the personality of the follower and the situation. The leader's personality also has an impact on his behavioral repertory (action flexibility) and on his skill in selecting appropriate communication behaviors.[8]

The leader's needs and his related potential for responding to a variety of external stimuli (perceptual capacities) affect his response to the many stimuli that confront him. The follower, the situation and its physical phenomenon, other individuals, groups, organizations, the broader cultural context, and goals provide the basis for these stimuli. The leader's needs and perceptual capacities, in relation to the quality and quantity of available stimuli, determine his range of perceptions (perceptual flexibility) and provide him with a basis for attempts to influence.

The leader's needs significantly determine what he can see or do in the course of his attempts to influence and have an impact on how he is perceived by the follower. He must then identify the perceptions he believes relevant and accurate to attain specific goals. This ability to determine the accuracy or correctness of perception has been termed *sensitivity* (social and nonsocial sensitivity). The leader needs to be socially sensitive to relevant needs, feelings, and motivations of the follower as well as be socially sensitive to particular groups, organizations, and a variety of goals. A sensitivity toward self has been considered a possible correlate of sensitivity toward others and of interpersonal effectiveness.

When initially confronted with an incident or situation and assessment factors he designates as goal-relevant, the leader has his *psychologic map* available, which provides a basis for action. He assesses followers and the situation before acting—forms a mental image of barriers and facilitating circumstances that bear on the desired goals of his leadership behavior. He visualizes the action pathways open to him and which he believes will lead to leadership effectiveness. The psychologic map is a combination of accurate and inaccurate notions regarding relevant and nonrelevant items. Again his personality comes into play in that his needs and his capacities for behavior (action capacities) determine his range of available communcation behaviors (action flexibility). Emphasis is placed on the leader's ability to communicate, his skill in transmitting meaning by using symbols, including the leader's behavior, which affect the follower's receptivity or block the meaning of what the leader transmits. Nonverbal communication is most important. The leader needs to be sensitive to relevant attitudes of the follower and he needs to assess correctly the follower's feelings, motives, and perception of others.[9]

Influence is exerted through the communication process, the aim of which is to bring about coincidence between the meaning of information input (the information transmitted by the communicator) and output (the meaning of information received by the communicator). The leader uses communication stimuli as tools to affect the perceptual-cognitive structures of followers. He selects from his communication behaviors that which he feels will motivate the followers toward a desired change in attitude and eventually toward desired behavioral changes. "Certain *communication behaviors* are therefore *judged appropriate* by the leader and selected, and others are *judged inappropriate* and *rejected*."[10] A measure of leadership effectiveness is the degree to which the behaviors selected are actually appropriate and succeed in moving the followers toward goal attainment.

Thus, leadership is viewed to be a process, a cyclical process, in that events at any step may be fed back to the leader so that modifications in behavior may be made and parts of the sequence can be altered.

Stogdill constructed a theoretical system of individual behavior and group achievement based on performance, interaction, and expectation. The assumptions underlying the theory are (a) human beings act, perceive, feel, and learn, and these experiences determine somewhat their behavior in relation to other persons; (b) a social order exists and its nature determines to some extent the behavior of individuals as well as the kinds of groups formed in a given culture; and (c) the nature of a group will be determined by the kinds of people who make up its membership as well as the social environment of which it is a part.[11]

A group is seen as an input-output system. To increase output it will be necessary to increase input energy and values. Performances, interactions, and expectations are considered behavior inputs and are attributes of individuals, singly and in interaction. The effects of these behavior variables in combination are exhibited in the form of role differentiation and performance, or in group structure and operations. Role structure and group operations are properties of the group and result from interrelated performances, interactions, and expectations of members. The end effects of these personal and interpersonal behaviors, mediated through group structure and operations, are exhibited in the form of group achievement. The different aspects of achievement are productivity, morale, and integration.[12]

Operations that define a group are the demonstration that an interaction exists; that it is an open system (exchanges members and values with its environment); that successive interactions maintain the identity of the system; and that the structure of the system is determined by the actions and reactions of its members.[13]

Performance is defined as a response that may be identified as one of the actions or reactions constituting the operations of an interaction system. It is any response perceived by other members as identifying the actor as a participant in the operations of a group. "An act exhibited by an individual is a performance if it identifies him as a member of a group." [14]

Stogdill states that group structure and operations are founded on a substructure of individual performance and interactions. "Expectation, defined as readiness for reinforcement, is a function of drive, the estimated probability of occurrence of a possible outcome, and the estimated desirability of the outcome." [15] A personal value system is a highly generalized set of expectations in which estimates of desirability are mutually confirmed, with little reference to estimates of probability and which serves as a referent or criterion for evaluating the desirability of alternative outcomes. "The degree of generalization among these value systems may be conceived as so great that they are reinforced by almost all relevant outcomes." [16]

The drive of its individual members and the reinforcement they give to each other's expectations relative to the goal to be reached gives a group its motive power.[17] The degree of freedom exhibited by a group and its members is related to the amount of structure and to the consistency with which expectations are reinforced. The structure of the system can be described in accordance with differential performances, interactions, and expectations of its members. The group can exert effects upon each member that will structure his expectations and interactions, and pattern his performance somewhat in conformity with the normative expectation of the group. "The position of a group member becomes differentiated from other positions by virtue of the fact that the member exhibits predictable patterns of performance which elicit predictable responses from other members." [18]

The more a member initiates actions that elicit responses and reactions from other members, the greater the extent to which he structures the interaction system. In turn, the difference between his position and that of the other group members increases. The status of a position within a group is the degree of freedom granted its occupant in initiating and maintaining goal direction and structure of the system relative to the status and functions of all other positions. The general nature of the contribution that its occupant is expected to make toward the accomplishment of the group defines the function of the position.[19]

An organized group, then, may be regarded as a complex system of overlapping and interacting input values, structures, operations, and output values, all of which are in constant balance, change, and counterbalance.[20] Members of high status within a group are permitted to perform some functions, which neither the group as a whole nor the various subgroups can perform.

Based on the theoretical considerations presented, it may be stated that leadership can be viewed as an interactional process through which the goals of a group or organization can be met. Incorporated in this process is the value of the individual, his needs, abilities, and performances, whether in the role of leader or that of follower. Communication is a means through which leadership is exerted and goals achieved. Through acts of communication, influence is exerted and changes take place in the attitudes of followers.

Stogdill concludes that leadership is the process of influencing the activities and efforts of an organized group toward goal setting and achievement.[21] Inherent in the leadership process, with its focus on goal determining, facilitating, influencing, and achieving, is decision making. The steps in the decision-making process have been delineated by Griffiths. "It can be seen that a decision is essentially a judicial proceeding—that is, a state of affairs is present and a judgment is made concerning it. The judgment is such as to influence the action that results from the decision. Action is implicit in a decision. The judgment is made so that a course of action will be influenced." [22] A decision-making process has been delineated and includes: (a) the recognition, definition, and limitation of the problem; (b) analysis and evaluation of the problem; (c) establishment of criteria by which a solution will be evaluated or judged as acceptable and adequate to the need; (d) collection of data; (e) formulation and selection of the preferred solution(s) which have been pretested; (f) activation of the preferred solution which includes programming and controlling the action followed by evaluation of the results and the process itself.[23]

The foregoing presentation of leadership theoretical considerations supports the concept that leadership is a process and further supports the study of leader behavior within the nursing situation. It lends support to the selection and development of leader behaviors that relate to the leader as a person, his relations with others in a group or task situation, and his ability to think, communicate, to decide, facilitate, and influence specified goal achievement applied to the nursing situation.

Gibbs summarizes the status of leadership theory by designating three leadership principles: (a) leadership is always relative to the situation in that it flourishes only in a problem situation and the nature of its role is determined by the goal of the group; (b) leadership is always directed toward some objective goal; (c) leadership is a process of mutual stimulation (a social interactional phenomenon) in which the attitudes, ideals, and aspirations of the followers play as important a determining role as do the individuality and personality of the leader.[24] Fiedler adds another dimension when he states that a systematic body of theory is essential not only for the sake of organizing the research findings in the field, but also to provide practical guidance in the selection, training, placement, and evaluation of leadership in the innumerable situations that require group effort. He points out three reasons why leadership research has not flourished as hoped. First, leadership research is plagued by a number of very difficult problems, one of which is that a large sample of comparable cases is difficult to find. Second, leadership phenomena turn out to be highly complex social processes requiring data that reflect and entail correspondingly complex statistical interactions. Finally, theory of leadership has not kept pace with empirical research in this area, with the major thrust in the field dating from the beginning of World War II.[25]

NURSING LEADERSHIP PROCESS

Leadership may occur within the formal organization and the latter is all the better if leadership is a companion process to administration, management, and supervision. However, leadership belongs to formal and informal organizations and is not bound by organizational boundaries. It can occur whenever, wherever, and with whomever there is need for goal setting and influence toward goal achievement by a person who is a leader and a person(s) who is led.

With this view in mind the authors have attempted to state a definition of leadership, designate the nursing leadership process, delineate specific behaviors inherent in the process, and determine the dimensions of the process.

The theoretical formulations about leadership provide a useful framework for thinking about, analyzing, synthesizing, and researching leadership further. Theoretical formulations in and of themselves have little value, however, unless they are put into action. In other words, the theories need to be operationalized for testing purposes and need to be applied to or serve as the basis for direct action.

The theoretical developments and the collective research related to leadership available at this time should give direction to the development of leadership for nursing, include a taxonomy of behaviors that would rightfully be labeled leadership behaviors, and what is known about leadership, generally, should be applied to nursing specifically.

Thus, the literature was searched for definitions of leadership. These were analyzed and other definitions developed which seemed clearer, more appropriate to research development relating to leadership at the present time, and which would be applicable to nursing.

For the purposes of this presentation, leadership is defined as the process of influencing the behavior of other persons in their effort toward goal setting and achievement. *Nursing leadership is a process whereby a person who is a nurse effects the actions of others in goal determination and achievement.* This implies the defining and planning for nursing in an interactional setting. *Nursing* is an encounter with a client and his family in which the nurse observes, supports, communicates, ministers, and teaches: She contributes to the maintenance of optimum health, and provides care during illness until the client is able to assume responsibility for his own basic human needs; when necessary, she provides compassionate assistance for the dying.

Inherent in the operational definitions is a grasp of the direction of change and the ability to determine the direction and extent of change as well as to utilize the humane and moral means (communication, reward, punishment, coercion, etc) followers accept as they pursue goal achievement. Failure to move or change means no goal achievement, no leadership, no followership.

As the survey and analysis of the literature progressed, it was necessary to go beyond the definition of leadership and nursing leadership so that available knowledge would have meaning for nursing. Direct application of theory to practice was the goal. If the process of leadership could be determined, a process that would enhance goal setting and ensure goal achievement, a major step would be achieved toward the implementation of available knowledge related to leadership. This process, when identified and developed, could be learned as are all other processes needed for the practice of nursing, ie, the nursing process, the research process, the teaching-learning process.

Available material in the literature on leadership and nursing leaders—including theories, definitions, opinions, behavior designations, expectations, etc.—were analyzed to determine if evidence of a process could be found. As the review continued, it became obvious that a few key words and phrases were dominant and that clusters of behaviors, thought to be leadership behaviors, were related to these key words and phrases. The consistency in the use of key words and phrases such as interaction, influence, guiding, satisfying individual and group needs, decision making related to goal determination and achievement, changing, communicating, providing, supported the contention that a process could be developed. Four key words were extracted from the words and phrases used most frequently. Most other frequently cited words and phrases related to one or another of these terms and seemed to be a dimension of or to flow from them. Terms could be clustered and categorized with a term selected to name the cluster.

The four key terms were *deciding, relating, influencing, and facilitating*. These terms were felt to be strategic to put into operation the definition of leadership and of nursing leadership, as defined earlier. A rereview of these terms satisfied the authors that these four terms were inclusive enough, with sufficient differences between and among them, to be of value. The sequence of the four terms was considered logical and useful.

After the components of the process were identified, the authors asked a sample group of senior baccalaureate nursing students ($N = 21$) and first- and second-year masters nursing students ($N = 104$) to respond to questions about these components. Respondents were asked if they perceived deciding, relating, influencing, and facilitating as essential to the nursing leadership process, and to rate the four component terms in order of priority. (See Appendix for full report, p. 200-214.) The authors' identification and ordering of the process components were supported by the respondents. All respondents agreed with the selection of process components and most supported the proposed ordering. Respondents were almost evenly divided as to placing deciding and relating as first in importance ($N = 46$ for deciding as first and $N = 47$ for relating as first). However, there was a clear distinction when responses were viewed in terms of ordering in the second place. Relating was clearly designed for second place ($N = 47$) in contrast to deciding ($N = 29$).

The nursing leadership process is a process through which determined goals are achieved through the four components of deciding, relating, influencing, and facilitating. Permeating all components is the act of communicating.

Participants in the nursing leadership process are the leader and the follower(s). Variables internal and external to the leader and follower(s) have an impact on goal determination and achievement when utilized in a nursing situation. Diagrammatically, the nursing leadership process is envisioned as demonstrated in Fig. 1.

Change occurs from the point of goal determination to the point of goal achievement. Feedback is needed to evaluate the realization of determined goals. Failure to meet the goals fully will reactivate the components deciding, relating, influencing, and facilitating as demanded by the situation to fully achieve the determined goal(s) (Fig. 2).

Power is inherent in the leadership process, as is flexibility to manipulate components and subcomponents to achieve maximum effect. Power is given to the leader as long as followers sanction this. Power is increased if goal determination and achievement are accomplished in an effective manner. Thus, no one type of leadership style is appropriate to all of nursing. The variations encountered in nursing situations, with differences in follower participants as well as in the degree and number of crises and the amount of available decision-making time, demands a flexible leadership style even in any one day. Also superimposed upon the process are short-term, intermediate, and long-range goals in the nursing situation. This

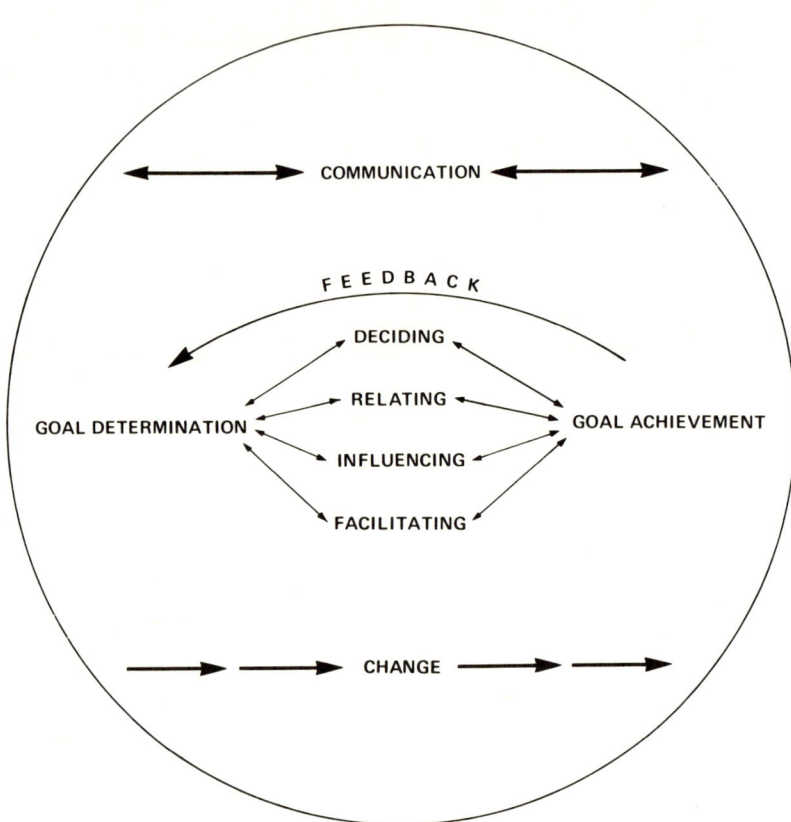

FIG. 1 Nursing Leadership Process.

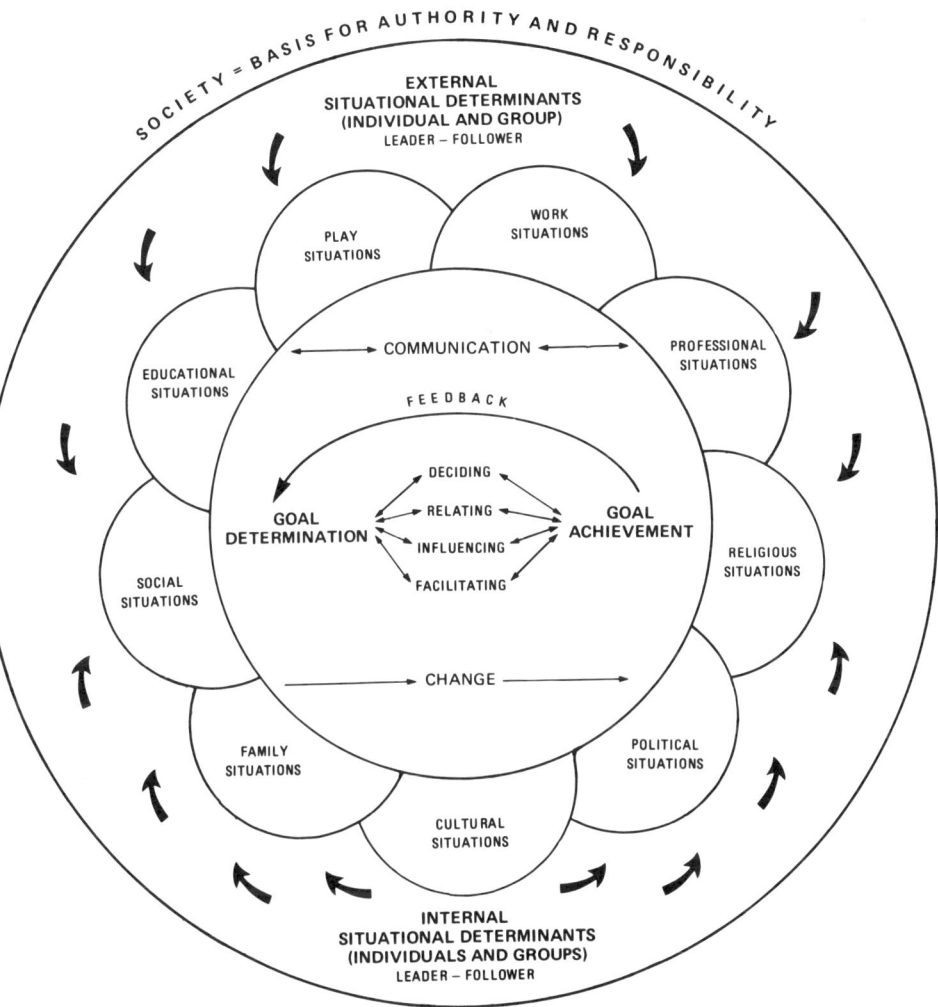

FIG. 2 Models of Nursing Leadership Process.

gives a multidimensional focus to utilization of the nursing leadership process. Change permeates the entire process from beginning to end. Change affects the participants and the situation, for neither is the same once the process becomes operative. The acts associated with the nursing leadership process are always in the direction of goal achievement. Thus, if goal determination is legitimate, appropriate, realistic, and moral and if the acts of deciding, relating, facilitating, and influencing are humane, are appropriate singly or in combination, are within the skill of the leader and acceptable, expected, and viewed as helpful by the follower(s), then it can be said that goal achievement will occur and the nursing leadership process is being effectively utilized.

The nursing leadership process is applicable with clients, well or ill, families, groups of clients and families, with peers and colleagues, and with special interest groups (consumer, health-related personnel, health professionals). The process is also applicable in the leader's immediate surroundings and with more distant groups —local, state, and national. It is possible to use the process despite a diversity of goals and even with diffuse goals that have a narrow and/or broad impact on those directly involved or who are touched or affected by goal achievement. An example of a broad impact would be the utilization of the nursing leadership process to achieve quality delivery of health and nursing service on a national level. Although the number of persons striving to achieve this goal is limited the results of goal achievement will affect every citizen, alien and visitor to the United States.

After the components of the nursing leadership process were identified, the human actions inherent in each were identified. These actions are called behaviors and their designation is termed a taxonomy of behaviors related to the nursing leadership process. Permeating each of the four processes of deciding, relating, influencing, and facilitating is the act of communicating. Communication, however, is not viewed as a separate component because it cannot be separated from the four identified components. It is inherent throughout the process because the process components are only realized through communication.

TAXONOMY OF BEHAVIORS RELATING TO NURSING LEADERSHIP PROCESS

Process Component—*Deciding*—Communicating is inextricably incorporated in this component

Behaviors

- analyzing
- assigning
- assuming
- choosing
- comparing
- concentrating
- concluding
- data collecting
- deducing
- delegating
- deliberating
- discerning
- disclosing
- discovering strategies
- discriminating
- distinguishing
- evaluating
- feeding back
- formulating
- guiding
- implementing
- informing
- inquiring
- judging
- measuring
- observing
- perceiving
- planning
- predicting
- probing
- responding
- risk taking
- seeking
- selecting
- setting precedent
- synthesizing
- validating

Process Component—*Relating*—Communicating is inextricably incorporated in this component

Behaviors

- appreciating
- arbitrating
- assisting
- attending
- bargaining
- behaving
- calming
- comforting
- concealing
- conversing

conveying
cooperating
criticizing
cutting off
differentiating
dignifying
directing
discriminating
effecting
enhancing
explaining
gossiping
greeting
ignoring
informing
interacting
  (a) approaching
  (b) initiating
  (c) continuing
  (d) terminating
  (e) withdrawing

listening
projecting
reacting
recognizing
reducing uncertainty
resisting
respecting
responding
revealing
sharing
socializing
speaking
supporting
sustaining
touching
transacting
understanding
using self
valuing
welcoming
withholding

Process Component—*Influencing*—Communicating is inextricably incorporated in this component

Behaviors

advancing
advocating
approving
assenting
brainwashing
censoring
challenging
choosing
coercing
comparing
competing
concealing
condemning

conditioning
condoning
confronting
controlling
convincing
credentialling
deceiving
deferring
demoting
detaining
dictating
directing
disapproving

discharging
disciplining
disclosing
disguising
dissenting
distinguishing
divulging
duping
elevating
framing
hiding
identifying
ignoring
impressing
indoctrinating
inducing
inspiring
internalizing
interpreting
legitimizing
managing
manipulating
modifying
moralizing
motivating
neglecting

obligating
ordering
pacifying
persuading
plotting
politicizing
praising
prodding
promoting
proving
punishing
reasoning
rejecting
rewarding
ruling
satisfying
secrecy
separating
socializing
subterfuging
suspending
teaching
tattling
telling
threatening

Process Component—*Facilitating*—Communicating is inextricably incorporated in this component

Behaviors

acquiring
altering
allocating
arranging
authorizing
balancing
bargaining

budgeting
causing
changing
claiming
closing
collecting
creating

demonstrating	performing
directing	potentiating
dispersing	preserving
distributing	providing
dividing	publishing
enabling	recording
freeing	reimbursing
getting	requesting
giving	requisitioning
involving	seeking
modifying	showing
monitoring	starting
negotiating	supervising
opening	surveying
organizing	tending
paving	utilizing

The style of nursing leadership will be determined by the behaviors demonstrated for each of the four components. Since the behaviors listed in the taxonomy indicate a large array of avilable behaviors, their precise utilization (and any additional behaviors to be identified through practice and research) will depend on the leader's personality and knowledge, the follower's receptivity, and the variables in the setting.

Effective or ineffective leadership will be designated according to the success with which determined goals are achieved. The level of success in leading must take into account nursing leadership behaviors inherent in deciding, relating, influencing, and facilitating.

To summarize—The dimensions of nursing leadership behavior can be illustrated diagrammatically, as indicated in Figure 3.

The authors created premises related to the nursing leadership process and applied the components of the process for illustrative purposes, thus indicating the ease with which the process may be utilized. Each premise is accompanied by a myth that is refuted. The premises serve as guiding principles in implementing the process.

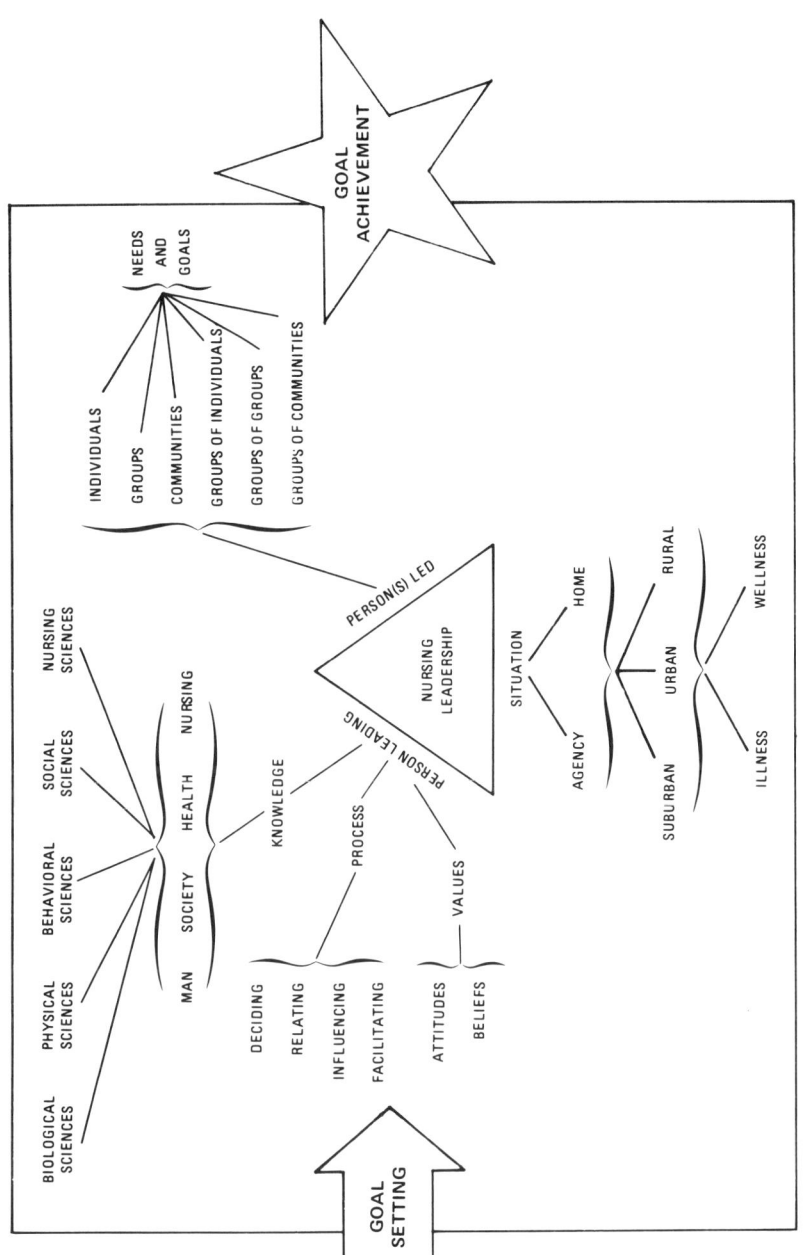

FIG. 3 Dimensions of Nursing Leadership.

Premise 1: To use the nursing leadership process, the nurse must have knowledge and skill.
Myth: A person is born to be a leader.

Factual knowledge from numerous disciplines is necessary if the nurse is to *inspire* the confidence and trust of her colleagues as well as the confidence of clients for whom she is caring. She also must have sufficient knowledge to ensure her own self-confidence. She needs to be convinced of her ability to develop her own framework so that she can determine why an event is occurring and whether she can cope with it effectively.

The *decision-making* phase of the nursing leadership process requires a sound basis for making judgments and this basis rests on the broad, inclusive knowledge and skills of the decider. When faced with more than one alternative in planning client care, the nurse must decide which is the best alternative or route to follow. The client, on a 1:1 caring plan, is involved with the nurse in the decision making. As the client asks questions and reveals problems he is facing, the nurse uses her knowledge and background experience to assist him and herself in making decisions about care. A wide range of assessment factors are explored and various plans may be possible, each of which must be considered to determine the best route for this client, at this time and in this situation. The nurse's knowledge will assist her in recalling scientific facts to guide decision making. For example, the diabetic client will require a much lower carbohydrate intake than the high carbohydrate diet of his previous pattern. Or, a person who tends toward midmorning hypoglycemia plans a carbohydrate–protein snack to ward off the untoward effects of such a metabolic incident.

When dealing with groups of nursing and health care personnel responsible for a group of hospitalized clients, the decision-making process becomes more complex. Not only does the nurse concern herself with the problems and needs of the client, his family, and significant others, but she also concerns herself with the problems and needs of members of the staff. Knowledge of human behavior becomes an important factor in dealing with groups of people, both clients and staff. An understanding of what to expect as well as how to deal with various behavior patterns, deciding what to do, and choosing one of several alternatives, is crucial to effecting the nursing leadership process.

The knowledge acquired by the nurse provides her with a base from which she determines the actual and potential problems of clients and the staff with whom she functions. Assessing these problems in light of her own abilities and strengths, she decides, sometimes alone, sometimes in collaboration with clients and/or staff, which is the best of several alternative routes to follow for the good of all.

Depending upon the persons involved in the situation and the problems identified, components of relating and influencing may change in priority or blend into components more difficult to separate precisely from each other than are other components of the nursing leadership process. One can argue that in order to influence, one must relate; and in order to relate, one must influence. Be that as it may, each can be separately analyzed and then transposed from a higher to a lower position, or vice versa, as need be.

Relating to others requires an ample degree of charity (love), feeling, and value for one's fellow man. Trust and respect for another, be he client or co-worker, are essential elements in establishing a relationship that is to be productive of good effects. It is important that this kindness (charity), trust, and respect enter into and permeate all negotiations and encounters between individuals relating to each other.

The nurse leader sees the client and treats him as a person who has abilities and rights, strengths and limitations, and who may be experiencing some temporary incapacity in one or several of these areas. In order to be of assistance to the client, the nurse communicates her respect for the client as an individual by word and manner. When the client senses such respect for his rights and feelings, he reciprocates, usually by extending the same degree of respect to the nurse.

The nurse leader, through her knowledge of human behavior, has established a sound basis for a good relationship by treating the client with respect.

In dealing with co-workers, whether peers, subordinates, or superiors, the same knowledge of human behavior applies. To function collaboratively for the benefit of clients and of staff, mutual trust and respect must permeate all endeavors. Through group efforts, the talents of each and all can be utilized so that the client benefits and the staff realizes satisfaction in worthwhile and productive efforts.

A sound knowledge of human behavior enables the nurse leader to provide a stable, good relationship between clients and personnel by establishing an atmosphere of mutual charity, trust, and respect for the abilities, strengths, and rights of each to the eventual benefit of the client and the satisfaction of personnel.

The knowledge necessary to carry out the *influencing* phase of the nursing leadership process should be constructive and broad. All of the knowledge used to make decisions and to relate to others is required for influencing. Positive influence is paramount so that the nurse leader is moving constructively and productively to benefit all. In her role of leader, the nurse may be able to exert influence because those who are following, whether client or staff, are doing so because of the nurse's role and not because of the directions or instructions she is giving. Knowledge about roles and status will help the nurse leader acquire insight into the client's and the staff's responses to her. The desirable effect of the nurse's leadership should be that the client sees her as a knowledgeable and capable health worker. Such knowledge proves to the client that the nurse can direct and guide him to achieve the health goal shared by both. Her role as leader is reinforced when the client sees the nurse as a person to respect not only because of her role but because of her knowledge and expertise in the health endeavors of both (client and nurse). The purpose of influencing, ultimately, is to establish plans of care and to set these plans in motion—to implement them. Through knowledge of resources, available personnel potential, achievable goals, the nurse can influence the client to set reasonable goals and help the client to seek resources and people who will be most beneficial to him.

Thus, a wide range of constructive knowledge and skill is crucial to the nurse leader influencing the client in his search for reasonable goals and helpful resources and personnel.

To *facilitate* the entire operation, the nurse leader must know that all other phases of the process are completed satisfactorily or at least as completely as possible at the moment. Only if decisions have been made as to the best route(s) to follow, if relationships have been established, and if appropriate influences are felt, can the total process be facilitated. If, on reflection, it is determined that one or part of any component has been insufficiently explored and/or implemented, then facilitation is delayed until such components are completed.

Knowledge of what has been accomplished between and among nurse leaders and clients, as well as what the potential accomplishment is in terms of goals and desired ends, will assist the nurse leader in effecting changes and adjustments to enhance the situation. By knowing how to use the abilities of clients and personnel, the nurse leader can facilitate movement and hopefully progress, by meeting the needs of clients, to a situation of stability and eventual total health.

The facilitation phase of the leadership process is effected when all other phases are moving well and constructively; the nurse leader acts as overseer and prime mover to ensure progress and stability to achieve a state of health for the client.

The extent of the impact of nursing leadership, the style and kind of leadership, and the effectiveness or ineffectiveness of leadership behaviors are determined through the utilization of the nursing leadership process and the number of persons participating. Degrees of complexity are determined by the quantity and quality of decisions; the method, kind, and quality of influence; the effectiveness of relating; the kind and amount of facilitation; the extent of goal determination; the amount of change needed to bring about goal achievement; the total number of individuals involved; and the number of communications needed among participants to achieve the goals set forth.

Premise 2: Nursing leadership process is an intellectual and interpersonal process.
Myth: Leadership depends upon personality.

As has been known for a long time, and as noted earlier, nursing leadership is not based on traits and personal characteristics alone, but includes situational aspects and considers followers. Although personality traits constitute important attributes for the leader, a combination of traits, including the values held by the leader, respect for others, respect for self, holding a valuing regard for the rights of people, and understanding basic human needs and human responses to multiple situations, constitutes behavioral expectations for the leader.

The stereotype of the leader as charismatic with physical characteristics that imply overpowering others is not supported by research or actual practice. Facility with intellectual skills as problem determination, solution designation, and problem resolution are far more likely to be sought by persons willing to be led in a specific situation. Structuring a situation through goal determination is more likely to be viewed positively by followers and most likely to result in goal achievement. Goal achievement is assured if individuals influenced by and toward designated goals have a stake in the determination of these goals. Decisions and choices permeate all elements of the leadership process. Communication is the vital dimension permeating deciding, relating, influencing, and facilitating—the nursing leadership process elements.

Since leadership requires two or more persons and cannot be achieved by one individual alone, interpersonal skills play a significant role in determining goals and in efforts toward achieving them. The relationship must be ongoing, with the leader sensitive to the thoughts, feelings, and needs of the followers. Sensitivity to one's impact on others is strategic, and the leader should be aware and open to behavioral indicators in followers to determine if the intended impact has been made. Skill in listening attentively for meaning and feeling, the judicious use of silence, realistic behavior in face-to-face situations with others, adapting behavior to meet differing and changing interpersonal situations are only a few of the skills needed by the leader. Other interpersonal skills include demonstrating sensitivity to the ways people communicate with each other, criticizing an act rather than an individual, explaining reasons for criticism, and demonstrating an awareness of the influence of personal and interpersonal factors on thoughts and actions.

The nursing leadership process abounds with the need for intellectual and interpersonal skills. Critical thinking and decision making, which must be evident, include assuming responsibility for action taken, based on the leader's decision; the ability to grasp essentials of a problem and to see alternative solutions; to select appropriate solutions; the ability to assess a complex situation and reduce it to its component parts; discriminating between relevant, irrelevant, essential, and accidental data; recognizing and locating resources necessary to solve a problem; the ability to predict the consequences of decisions; demonstrating the ability to grasp ideas fully; and manifesting a mastery of known theories and knowledge pertaining to nursing.

Thus, although getting the job done—goal achievement—may reflect no leadership activity at all and may, in fact, be more in keeping with routine and/or automatic actions, it must truly be steeped in deciding, relating, influencing, and facilitating.

Stogdill points out that leadership is more likely a working relationship among members of a group through which a leader acquires active participation and demonstrates his capacity to carry cooperative tasks to completion rather than a matter of passive status or mere possession of a combination of traits. "Significant aspects of this capacity for organizing and expediting cooperative effort appear to be intelligence, alertness to the needs and motives of others, and insight into situations, further reinforced by such habits as responsibility, initiative, persistence, and self-confidence."[26] It is further pointed out that singular characteristics hold little leadership predictive significance. Stogdill summarizes by stating that the leader is characterized by a strong drive for responsibility and task completion, vigor and persistence in pursuit of goals, venturesomeness and originality in problem solving, drive to exercise initiative in social situations, self-confidence and sense of personal identity, willingness to tolerate frustration and delay, willingness to accept consequences of decision and actions, readiness to absorb interpersonal stress, ability to influence other persons' behavior, and capacity to structure social interactions systems to the purpose at hand.[27] These characteristics are mainly intellectual and interpersonal in nature.

Nursing leadership is expected to be a multifaceted role, ie, the leader relates to and serves as leader to a number of groups simultaneously. She is likely to be a leader for staff, a leader for nursing when relating to other publics, and a leader among nurse leaders on local, state, and national levels. Thus a broad range of intellectual and interpersonal skills is required. In summarizing the results of studies related to leader-follower interactions, Stogdill concludes that the leader may be required to "thread her" way with considerable discrimination so that her followers will work with her as a cohesive group. "The interaction patterns of superiors influence not only the interaction patterns of subordinates, but also their work and the kinds of problems they have to solve."[28] In addition, it was found that leaders differ from followers in their ability to initiate and sustain interaction with a wide range of personalities.[29]

Further, it is expected that the leader stimulates spontaneity in others, widens their field of participation, and expands the area of group freedom for decision and action. The leader "protects the weak and underchosen, encourages less capable members, is tolerant of the deviate, and accepts rather than rejects a wide range of member personalities."[30]

Thus, intellectual and interpersonal skills are strategic to effect and operationalize goal determination. Although personality traits are useful and important, personality alone is not the determining factor in goal achievement. Leadership involves intellectual, interpersonal, and technical (social, administrative, managerial, political) skills which enable the leader to maintain group cohesiveness and the drive and productivity held valuable by the group or organization with whom she functions.[31] It also helps if the leader possesses a high degree of task motivation and personal integrity.

> *Premise 3:* Nursing leadership implies mastery over ignorance and mastery of goals by *working with* people, but not mastery *over* people.
> *Myth:* A leader must be overpowering and aggressive to make an impact.

Perhaps the most striking requirement for the nursing leader is the development and display of intellectual skills. Intellectual skills include critical thinking, problem solving, making sound judgments, validating inferences, predicting the success of solutions, developing appropriate solutions—including solutions that set a precedent—

accommodating large amounts of data, ordering data, searching for data required to complete the data base, categorizing, comparing, synthesizing, and analyzing data, demonstrating foresight into future needs and goals based on knowledge of what was, what is, and what could and should be. Determining the timing of strategies, delegating strategies; choosing the right person for the right situation, evaluating one's knowledge base; and seeking the knowledge and information needed to make purposeful, accurate, and astute decisions, are additional intellectual skills.

Everyone makes many decisions every day, ranging from when to get out of bed in the morning to when to go to bed at night. Not only does the leader make decisions, but the decisions she makes have an impact on others as well as herself. Decisions made for others are important and must be considered seriously. To refrain from making a decision is a major decision. Decisions may be those made previously and found to work well, they may be modifications of prior decisions, or they may include precise decisions as to when a particular decision will be implemented as in policy making and effecting. Thus, there are decisions about decisions, choices, abstaining from decision making, precise timing for a decision, and the decision to foster a climate most conducive to implementing a decision.

Decision making by itself is insufficient, however. Decision making must be coupled with the ability to relate. Relating, too, incorporates decision making. With whom shall one relate, for what purpose, what opening, what conversation, what communication techniques would be most helpful, what needs do people express and/or have, what knowledge must the nurse have about an individual's age, life style, sociocultural and economic background in order to facilitate working with people, are but a few questions involved in decisions about relating.

Being comfortable with one's self and refraining from using a situation to meet one's own neurotic needs are expected if one is to work with people effectively and successfully. The nurse leader must have a broad knowledge of man, society, health, and nursing. She must be a student of human behavior, of the communication process, and of the group process. She must know how to relate to a broad range of persons whose goals, aspirations, beliefs, yearnings, life styles, view of health and illness may be quite different from hers.

She needs a broad knowledge of man so that she can anticipate these factors when urging persons to set goals and work to achieve stipulated goals.

The nurse leader must have a view of the future. Failure to look at the future and to be unaware of external and internal influences that have an impact on nursing and a bearing on nursing practice—of how and where it takes place, who will practice nursing, and how much is paid for it and by whom—are detrimental to any attempt at leading. To lead means to be out in front. Favoring the status quo and ignoring the reason for the existence of nursing—to meet the health and nursing needs of the citizens—is regressive and out of tune for both leaders and followers.

Looking back has merit for it helps one gain insight into the why and the outcome of earlier decisions, particularly those that affect the present. The present is the time for implementing new decisions, decisions that soon will be recorded as past. Thus, the future must allow for foresight, and for the designation and the planning so needed to ensure that preferred changes occur rather than those thrust upon us or for which nursing was either not ready or for which present or past decisions made little or no difference.

To permit ignorance and ineffectiveness to continue in nursing education and nursing services dooms us to failure and eventual extinction. Effective changes in the nursing care system occur only through and with people. The more encompassing and broad the change, the greater the number of persons—citizens, nurses, other health workers—involved. These people must be involved by free choice, not by mastery over others. Changes in the health care system can be singular, multiple, and varied. Some will be minor and others will or must be major. In all, a nurse leader with the necessary knowledge about man, society, health, and nursing will be in the forefront if her followers—citizens, nurses, other health workers—give her the opportunity to lead based on her ability to work cooperatively and collaboratively with people to determine goals and achieve them.

Premise 4: Nurse leaders are able to develop and utilize intelligent followers.
Myth: Intelligent people are not followers.

Studies have proven that intelligence, adjustment, and extroversion are highly significant to leadership. Persons of intelligence who are extroverted will attract similar persons. Leadership requires a leader–follower coalition for effectiveness. Research indicates that good followers are more like leaders and may develop into leaders. Followers are seen as members of a leadership team, even though their own personal influence over others may be undetectable.

The leader's task is complicated. It requires production through general agreement and decisions that will be strictly accepted and carried into action by those whose interests are involved. Therefore, followers must be intelligent. A leader has unearthly force, vision, personal magnetism, scorns fear of the unknown and untested. The leader is enterprising, ingenious, courageous, and determined. It takes an inordinate amount of knowledge and intelligence to be a leader, to identify followers, and to follow a leader.

General trends indicate that leadership status is associated with superior intelligence. The combined and applied intelligence of leader and follower, rather than level of intelligence of either per se, are important in cooperative productive behavior toward goal achievement. Contributions and communications must be understandable to and must be in accordance with the thoughts of contemporaries if one is to rise to a position of leadership.

In summary the nursing leadership process encompasses the four dimensions: deciding, relating, influencing, and facilitating which require that leaders and followers be intelligent beings. Persons of intelligence are needed to decide upon and achieve goals. Leaders must be intelligent to maximize and utilize the abilities of group members. Followers must be intelligent to recognize persons who can show the way and lead.

Premise 5: Successful nursing leadership depends upon mutual stimulation of leader and follower.
   Myth: Motivation of the leader is less important than is motivation of the follower.

Each situation in nursing is a person-oriented encounter. Some of the people involved are the providers of care, that is, they provide services. Others involved in nursing are the clients, the recipients of care; they are the persons who are in need of or require some services.

The goal of each nursing situation has as its ultimate aim a number of secondary purposes that are tangential to or spin off from the primary goal. For all persons to move forward progressively toward goal attainment, there must be some order in the group. To achieve this order, leader and followers become an inherent part of each group involved in nursing. A leader can exist only if at least two persons are involved. Without at least one follower there can be no leader. Without a leader, there is no one to follow.

In any setting in which nursing is to take place, the leader may, and usually is, involved with more than one follower, but the number of followers in any one situation varies widely. The reason for a leader–follower situation is to accomplish certain ends for the clients with whom nurses are functioning. If they are to function as a cohesive group of workers, certain elements must be inherent in the work situation. One very important element is mutual stimulation.

The significance of mutual stimulation is that each member of the group must experience motivation and satisfaction if client goals are to be achieved. Motivation of the follower suggests that this group of persons is involved with the work process in such a way that each feels he is an essential part of the group effort. Ideas and suggestions contributed by all group members act as sources of support and encouragement for the client. By understanding the client's problems and needs the group of followers learns the direction their activities should take. As they see the client deriving some benefit from the group effort, each member feels he has contributed to the total effort made to achieve client-set goals. When the client is too ill to be involved in the process, the group members involve the client's family or significant others from whom data are gathered to help all group members recognize the client's needs.

The total group of nurses, leaders, and followers act as stimulators and motivators for the client. Within the working group, each individual, which includes the leader and the follower, needs to be recognized. Each must be able to function in a supportive environment, with appropriate recognition for successful endeavors, and with the opportunity for self-development. The leader needs to know that she has accurately appraised the needs of the staff just as the entire group needs to know they were on target in assessing the client needs.

The personal needs of the leader will be different from those of the staff because she not only occupies a different role, that of leader, but is also an individual. Each individual in the group exhibits his or her own personality, character, and needs, because no two individuals are alike; each is unique.

The basic principle of motivation necessary for job satisfaction applies to each member of the group, no matter what role each plays within the group.

As the numbers of groups increase, and as each group increases in size, basic needs for motivation and stimulation increase in number and in intensity, but the needs are not eliminated.

To enhance motivation for all persons in the nursing situation, several components are essential to group functioning. The leader has the major responsibility for effecting these, but essentially the leader as well as the client benefits. A positive atmosphere, or a climate conducive to stimulation, is important to motivate the nurse and the client. Coordination of the many, varied activities that are part of helping, living, and communicating with all persons involved in goal-directed actions, opportunity for reflection, and earned rewards are necessary for the continued stimulation and encouragement of group members.

Premise 6: The ordering of components of the nursing leadership process change according to the goals to be achieved, the abilities of group members, and the environmental influences on activities taking place.

Myth: Components of the nursing leadership process are specifically ordered and must be pursued before the nurse leader can proceed to the next component.

Within this premise there are three themes: (a) the nursing leadership process consists of certain definable components or parts; (b) specific factors determine the extent to which any one component is needed and when; (c) responsibility for implementing the nursing leadership process lies with a group of professional persons, among whom there is at least one leader and one or more followers.

The essence of any activity is movement, ie, action or progress. In moving toward a goal, certain motions and behaviors can be defined grossly and superficially, or they can be analyzed precisely and carefully according to the angles, speed, contours, characteristics, or essence of each part of the behaviors that becomes a total force to accomplish a goal. The behaviors deciding, relating, influencing, and facilitating can be analyzed and examined.

At the present time, nursing is performed by a group of nurses who are striving to help the client achieve his health care goals. Within this group, one of the nurses is the leader and the others are followers. The client is usually perceived as a member of a group, all of whom are directing their efforts toward the client's health care goals.

The point at which the group enters the nursing leadership process will depend upon the perceptions of its members and the specific goals they have in mind. The characteristics of the group members will determine the degree of emphasis directed to the relating phase at the outset of the activity. As progress is made in establishing working relationships among nursing personnel and client, influencing actions will appear among group members. This may take place before there is any attempt at decision making. Having accomplished certain ends, facilitation may then be initiated by some members; simultaneously, other members may be involved in the decision making, relating, and influencing stages for various purposes and with varying degrees of success.

Analysis of such goal pursuits reveals that no one phase can be isolated from the others, and that the separation of each phase for discussion is primarily academic. In the actual practice of the nursing leadership process the phases seem to blend into a whole or total unit.

Because nursing is concerned with service to persons in need, the activities of nursing must be adjusted and adapted to changes that occur in the client. The moods, physiologic needs, emotional components, and spiritual demands of the client can change in a brief span of time. To steer the nursing group in the direction most helpful to the client, the nurse needs to be tuned to communications from the client. This may necessitate rapid movement among each phase of the nursing leadership process so that some activities may overlap; that is, some phases may be operative concurrently.

An additional dimension among the workers is the potential change in personnel among the group. Just as the needs of the client can change in a brief period of time, so, too, the needs of group members can change; flexibility and ready adaptability are required of all, especially the nurse leader. The leader of the group must have a keen sense of members' abilities and strengths. Matching these traits with the client's needs at any given moment is a primary task of the nurse leader. Throughout such a process, the nurse leader uses the nursing leadership process in a very precise, deliberate, and careful manner. The dimension of leading a group of nursing personnel, plus that of leading a group of clients is a multifaceted challenge, kaleidoscopic in nature.

Just as the sun influences life on earth, so will the environment in which nurses and clients are found influence their behavior and actions. Although precise predictions are not possible, there is a potential for speculating how certain behaviors will surface. For instance, a group of workers may be more positively responsive to directions on a bright, sunny day than on a dreary, rainy day. A well-rested person, free from serious personal worry, will be able to devote more attention to the problems of others than one who is fatigued and burdened with concerns outside the client situation. A hospital setting in which employees feel free to use initiative will produce a different type of client care than one that is too severely bound to policies "sent down" from higher echelons. A client's home may provide him (the client) with much more ease and comfort than the strange environment of a hospital. Each of these climates produces a different setting for client and nurse, and hence is a different challenge to the nursing leadership process.

Although there are individual preferences about whether one prefers to function as a group member or alone, there are advantages to the group endeavor. Built into the activities of a group are (a) the sharing of ideas and (b) the evaluation of ideas. An idea is usually generated by one person; it may be suggested by a group follower or a group leader. In any case, many ideas are only partial ideas; when presented for group discussion, this idea can be developed into a creative complete idea the group can then put into action. A positive outcome of such an exercise is that everyone has contributed to the total group effort and each person feels motivated to implement action.

Though subjectivity is valuable in reflecting on ideas and actions, there is benefit in objective evaluation, too. Functioning alone prohibits group evaluation of goals set and actions performed. With group members available for review, a constant check is at hand to ensure that gaps are filled and needs are not neglected.

Premise 7: The nursing leadership process is applicable to individuals and groups.
Myth: The application of the leadership process is always the same.

The leadership process is continuous and remains constant in its application and utilization. However, the degree to which each of the components is applied varies with the complexity and the number of variables in the situation. Leadership centers on a situation. Leadership between individuals and groups always follows movement toward achievement of a mutually accepted goal.

There was a time, celebrated in sagas, stories, ballads, and songs, when leadership was entrusted to a leader. The number of leaders was small, their knowledge limited, their expertise primitive, the range of their involvement narrow, and the reach of their power marginal and confined by set boundaries. But these celebrated persons were always completely in charge.

The increase in man's territory and number and the overabundance of knowledge, technology, and modernization has made the vertical society obsolete. Leadership is now one to one, one to a few, one to many, and many to many. Leadership may also be vertical or horizontal. However, the complex needs of society and our dependence on many, rather than one, require that leadership becomes horizontal as well as vertical.

The process of leadership remains the same whether the leader deals with one, a few, or many followers. Elements of deciding, relating, influencing, and facilitating are required to decide upon and achieve goals, whether one deals with an individual, group, community, or nation. The key to the leadership of many is inherent in the leader's application of its elements. Although only one person makes the decision, followers help the leader decide. An idea originates only in one person's mind, no matter how that idea is improved upon, elaborated, and refined.

Premise 8: Nursing leadership is more involved and complex as the number of interacting persons increases.

Myth: Effective leadership requires a controlled number of followers.

Chester Barnard points out that the complexity of the relationship in any group increases very rapidly as the number of persons in the group increases. For example, if there are two persons in the group, there is one relationship, whereas for a five-person group there are 10 relationships. The number of relationships increases rapidly to 45 for a 10-person group, 105 for a 15-person group and jumps to 1225 for a 50-person group.[32]

Jay points out that ". . . although an idea can originate in one person's mind, it can be greatly improved if six or seven people question and add to it, elaborate on and refine it, in the same way—six or seven people are much better at evaluating it than one."[33] He indicates that the major advantages are size and the variety of ideas that come from a team. When an idea is only a half idea, team members may produce the other half as part of their collective action.[34]

Jay proposes that a 10-member group is the most effective and that often large groups are composed of multiple 10-member groups. He also feels, though, that in terms of group size, if the group works effectively, then regardless of its size it contains the right number of members.[35] Jay predicts that corporation managers will soon find that their major task will be the support and development of effective 10-member groups to insure morale and the long-range future of their organization. "It may be a difficult switch, but there is a powerful force operating on their side: the ten-groups are trying to form themselves all the time." [36]

The nursing leadership process can be applied to individuals and groups, but becomes more involved and complicated as the complexity and number of variables in the situation increases. Not only is communication more complex as the number of individuals increases, but great demands are placed on the leader to coordinate human activity directed toward goal achievement. Goals to be achieved may be singular or multiple. The status of the leader's role, ie, whether in the emerging leader role, or as status leader for a preexisting group, reveals another variable that must be considered. In nursing, situations with any or all of these dimensions prevail, and it is not unusual to expect an individual leader to function in emerging roles with some groups, to organize others for goal designation and achievement purposes, to lead an established group of individuals, and to participate with other nurse leaders, health care leaders, community leaders, state and national leaders to accomplish a myriad of goals, related and unrelated.

The leader must realize that she is required to function with varied groups for multiple purposes, with inherent demands for deciding, relating, influencing, and facilitating and develop physical, psychic, and moral strength. Whether simple or complex, the elements of the leadership process remain constant. The application of these elements, the timing, the ordering, the level emphases placed on certain components or elements of components at specific and varying times depend on the requirements for leadership demands in a situation.

Premise 9: Leadership is a concept in itself, separate and distinct from administration, management, and supervision.
Myth: All administrators, managers, and supervisors in nursing are nursing leaders.

Of the major terms in the premise, the Webster and Oxford Dictionaries define only the term leadership distinctly, thus indicating that administration, management, and supervision are synonymous. Leadership is different and unique from administration, management, and supervision. The terms in the premise are not interchangeable. Many persons inappropriately call administrators, managers, and supervisors leaders. Webster defines the terms as follows: leadership means to lead or show the way; administration is management; management is the act of handling, controlling or directing, and supervision is designated as directing or managing.[37, 38]

Management, supervision, and administration are the methods by which policies are implemented to meet organizational goals determined by others. They are the tools used to achieve a goal. In no way can management, supervision, and administration be equated with leadership. However, leadership and leaders may utilize management, supervision, and administration within the leadership process. Influence and power positions within a social organization are constantly referred to as positions of leadership. Nurse administrators, managers, and supervisors are often called leaders, but they are only leaders if and when they know and can implement all components of the nursing leadership process.

The nursing leadership process, ie, deciding, relating, influencing, and facilitating, is required in order to decide upon and to achieve goals. These dimensions are not found in their entirety in either administration, management, or supervision. Only some elements of the leadership process, not all, are found in each.

Nurse administrators, managers, and supervisors carry out decisions and policies of others, who are the goal deciders. In most formal institutions and organizations, goal determination and achievement occur through a variety of persons and groups at different levels, but only one person or group carries out the total process. Only a leader or leaders implement the total nursing leadership process. Administration, management, and supervision utilize techniques that split the process according to hierarchic arrangements—either vertically, horizontally, or a combination of both.

Jay states that "The Macavity system is only a symptom of a much deeper reluctance to talk about leadership or accept it or admit that it happens."[39] Macavity system of management is a term invented by Jay and applied to situations (management or leadership) when it is impossible to identify the person(s) responsible for decisions affecting others. He goes on to say that elegant euphemisms are utilized to avoid saying that someone is a leader. Management, administration, and supervision are frequently the euphemisms employed. The fact must be faced that there is a nursing leadership process that people—actual human beings—must exercise and that leadership is neither administration, nor management, nor supervision.

Nurses and nursing must cease and desist evading and accept the fact that each professional nurse must be a leader and must be taught the nursing leadership process. No longer can the "Macavity" system be used for escape. Nor can nurses continue to use, in nursing care, only the tools of leadership, ie, administration, management, or supervision, instead of implementing the nursing leadership process, ie, goal determination and achievement through deciding, relating, influencing, and facilitating.

Nurses must learn and implement the nursing leadership process in conjunction with the nursing process to provide care. Only by applying the nursing leadership process can the professional nurse lead or show the way in nursing.

Premise 10: Nursing leaders are predominantly women.
Myth: All leaders are men.

The premise that nursing leaders are predominantly women, but not exclusively so, is supported by the most up-to-date knowledge relating to leadership, as situationally determined. Early theorists, writing on leadership, sought to account for the emergence of leadership by examining qualities of the leader or elements in the leadership environment. The interaction between individual and situation is the way leadership is explained today. Characteristics of the individual and the demands of the situation interact in a manner that demand the leadership status be assumed.

For centuries nursing has been traditionally an occupation open to women. The art of nursing is strongly tied to comforting and supporting. These acts are closely allied to mothering, and, in the order of this universe, mothers are females. There is and always has been a predominance of women in nursing, because the situation attracted them. Since the occupation was almost exclusively filled with women, the leaders who emerged were women. Therefore, the majority of leaders in nursing are women.

In is interesting that statistics indicate that, although few in number, a large percentage of male nurses are employed in top administrative positions in nursing. In a 1914 text titled *Training School Methods and the Head Nurse,* Charlotte Aikens wrote that competent male nurses were prepared by hospitals to overcome the inefficiency of the average hospital orderly in the care of male patients. Aikens stated that "the young man's field is more limited as a nurse than that of the young woman, considering that he will hardly be called on to assume charge of a hospital or to become a head nurse." [40] In 1975 male nurses are employed in the field of nursing as head nurses, instructors, professors, deans of nursing programs, directors of nursing services, and as executives in national nursing organizations. Nursing is an occupation that has nothing to do with gender.

Two dimensions in the nursing leadership process considered to be strong female traits are relating and facilitating. Dominance and aggression (negative traits in leadership) are considered unfeminine. Certain antithetical psychologic qualities are routinely paired off sexually. Men are said to be active, aggressive, analytic and autonomous; women are passive, peaceful, intuitive, and social. Four sex differences have been fairly well established. Girls have greater verbal and interpersonal abilities. Girls excel in social goals; boys excel in visual-spatial ability and move ahead in mathematic skills. Boys are more aggressive, where aggressiveness is defined as involving the intent of one person to injure another. There is no consistent sex difference in psychologic and intellectual qualities. Such differences are not demonstrable. The sexes do not differ in cognitive style or skills and cognition is essential in leadership.

A number of relationships appear to exist between an individual's personality and leadership status in groups. Dominance and interpersonal sensitivity are found to be positively related to leadership, whereas conservatism is negatively related. Evidence is available indicating that the relationship between personality factors and leadership varies with the technique of measuring the leadership used.

Findings suggest that leadership is independent of aggression or dominance or the mere possession of some combination of traits or personality. Rather, it appears to be a working relationship of a group in which the leader acquires status through active participation and by demonstrating the capacity to carry cooperative tasks through to completion. One does not become a leader by virtue of particular traits, characteristics, or gender, but rather by possessing attributes which by virtue of their relevance to the situation, are situationally determined by the other group members. This then establishes the relationship between leader and follower. The need for nursing care is the situation. The leader is the nurse, the provider of nursing care. The client is the recipient and participant in goal determination and achievement.

Premise 11: Nursing leaders care about clients and contribute to nursing service.
Myth: Assuming the role of leader in nursing removes the nurse from the client.

Nursing is performed in a variety of settings. The term *nursing service* usually suggests an acute care setting, where organized nursing services are provided by different levels of personnel. In such a setting, where various types of nursing personnel are employed, the professional nurse is the nursing leader. However, this is not limited to setting. The professional nurse is the one responsible for directing the activities of other nursing employees and is responsible for the care provided for the client in each and all environments.

In order to ensure quality care for the client, the nurse assumes various roles in a variety of settings and one role is that of teacher. To teach the client, the professional nurse assesses the client's needs to determine his learning needs. Such assessment requires direct contact with the client; hence the professional nurse must maintain close association with the client.

Providing care, or ensuring a setting in which care can be provided, is one of the major purposes of the nurse, no matter in what situation or climate the client is located. There are numerous secondary purposes of nursing. When the professional nurse teaches the client about coping with his needs, one of the secondary purposes is achieved, that of contributing to nursing service. Ultimately, both goals or aims are necessary to accomplish nursing and client care, yet each can be identified separately and viewed on a primary and a secondary level.

In the process of teaching clients, the nurse has been accomplishing a direct and primary purpose for the benefit of the client. Secondarily, the nurse has been setting an example for other levels of nursing personnel. It behooves every nurse to demonstrate, by example, the activities and roles of nursing so that others can emulate them. Ancillary persons need such a model of nursing in order to know what "good nursing" is. In everyday situations, such role modeling is required to be a constant reminder to all personnel that "this is quality nursing." Setting such a model enables ancillary nursing personnel to set aims and goals that will probably require just a bit more than ordinary effort to achieve, but will be a stimulus to remind them that there are ever higher goals for which to strive.

The role modeling of the nursing leader is important for the professional staff nurses who function as part of the group of nursing personnel. This group needs encouragement, support, and stimulation; none of these needs is unique or peculiar to such a group of nurses; all are essential for any group of persons who work in a service capacity, merely because they are human. Providing such stimuli through role modeling is the nurse leader's responsibility.

Only if the nurse is aware of and alert to the needs of clients and those of personnel responsible for client care, can the professional nurse perform her role of model and teacher. In order to know these needs and to accurately assess them, the nurse leader must have pertinent and meaningful contacts with clients and with personnel. This responsibility implies a relative ease and confidence in the client situation and first-hand knowledge about the various facets of client care.

An added benefit derived from the nurse leader performing as a role model is the image of nursing projected to and perceived by the client. As the nurses engage in the activities of nursing effective in meeting client needs, the client perceives nursing at its best. This conveys to the public, client, and family, the role nursing assumes as a member of the health team. An important outcome of such modeling is that it provides information about the role of nursing, and also sets the stage for a more compatible common ground from which nurse and client can proceed to set goals of care. Ultimately, both nurse and client benefit from such role modeling and this serves as a base or foundation from which much constructive progress can proceed.

The following example illustrates a productive role-modeling situation. In an acute care setting, one of the events with which personnel must cope is that of the death of a client. This event presents many and complex challenges for the nurse and for the family. In a selected situation, one of the most effective ways to teach others to cope with the care of the dying person is to provide that care to the person; this includes demonstrating listening skills, extending empathy, physical and emotional support, and meeting specific requirements of the person who is dying. The skill of providing all of these aspects of care can be observed by those who are less experienced and less secure in administering care in such a demanding situation. This is truly a leader role fulfillment, a real challenge to the leader, but a satisfying activity when performed successfully. To show another nurse the appropriate way to cope with the dying client and to help the client's family are paramount roles of the nurse leader.

Premise 12: The effective utilization of the nursing leadership process requires a working knowledge of the nursing and research processes.

Myth: A non-nurse can effectively utilize the nursing leadership process.

One of the most complex factors in working with people is that of communication. Whether via the spoken or written word, or by signs or symbols, by facial expressions, or body language, in any variety of forms, communication poses major and continuing challenges to everyone.

To reflect upon the effective use of the nursing leadership process suggests a variety of dimensions. The controlling variable in the statement is the word "effective." This adjective adds a dimension of quality performance that essentially says: this is more than ordinary; it is superb, above average. Inherent within this idea is the suggestion that there are levels of performance and levels of quality that can be described as one performs the nursing leadership process. Although the nurse can decide, relate, influence, and facilitate in any and all situations, she may not be using the nursing leadership process effectively in all situations. This is not to say that she is not performing nursing actions; she is performing nursing but not as effectively or on the level necessary to be labeled the nursing leadership performance.

Having a working knowledge of the nursing process and of the research process suggests that the nurse must have more than a superficial knowledge of what nursing is all about. She must be able to act, to perform, to carry out all phases of these two separate and distinct processes, yet integrate the processes into all her activities; a large order, yes, but a necessary ingredient if the nurse is to use the nursing leadership process effectively.

The nursing process is essentially a problem-solving process: it is the knowledge of nursing and the use of this knowledge in solving client problems that makes the nursing process unique and distinct.[41] One solves problems continually in all experiences of life. Specific knowledge about the problem area makes each problem individual and distinctive. Only if the nurse knows what to look for in client assessment is she able to exercise appropriate judgment in setting priorities, plan soundly, to effect nursing action, and evaluate carefully. By the deliberate pursuit of these phases, nursing is accomplished.

The nurse needs knowledge about nursing to accomplish the nursing process and she needs sound knowledge about the nursing process to accomplish the nursing leadership process. An integral part of both the nursing leadership and the nursing process is the research process. Resolving client problems is an everyday challenge in nursing. The habitual pursuit of data collection for this purpose becomes second nature to the successful nurse. She has learned through experience that certain behaviors, certain patterns of acting, lead the way to success, to the accomplishment of a purpose, to the achievement of goals, and to the results sought. In many situations, this is entirely adequate. In some situations, however, this usual pattern is inadequate, if not of sufficient depth to meet the needs of some clients. Creativity and a different behavior become essentials in some situations and to meet the challenge the nurse must use the research process. Throughout the research process, the nurse follows approximately the same steps as in the problem-solving or nursing process, but rather than simply solve the problem after collecting data about the troublesome area, the nurse manipulates the data, examining and analyzing it from a variety of viewpoints, and reaches conclusions that suggest a different way of attacking the problem or of behaving or acting. This is the beauty of nursing—to provide the creative nurse with the opportunity to use all of her talents and all of her abilities, to benefit the clients. Through the judicious use of the nursing and research processes, the effective nurse, rather than the nonnurse, uses the nursing leadership process. The decisions made are of a qualitative nature, the relationships established are profitable to all concerned, the influencing activities are constructive and positive, and the facilitation is productive to goal achievement. All of these actions lead to the desired outcome—quality performance—the service product for which all consumers are crying and all nurses are striving.

> *Premise 13:* The most effective, efficient, and expeditious way to prepare persons who can implement the nursing leadership process is by acquiring a baccalaureate degree in nursing and further education through a graduate program in nursing.
> *Myth:* Nursing leaders are produced in every kind of educational program.

Leadership is a process which, like all others, has to be learned by gaining the required knowledge and then implementing it. The proper application of the leadership process is based on knowledge, expertise, skill, judgment, assessment, responsibility, and evaluation. Too many people in official leadership positions in nursing are there by default and because the situation made it necessary to name leaders, whether or not they possessed special educational preparation.

Education for leadership begins at the baccalaureate level in nursing and continues through graduate, continuing, and in-service education for as long as a person holds a position of responsibility in nursing.

A leader's unique function is to consolidate a large number of principles and accumulated knowledge and skills into policy and goals that extrude viable action. This requires a steady sense of direction, consultation with others, unremitting toil, unrewarded homework, and a willingness to forego ego trips. Leading is more than merely deciding and announcing that which is right and appropriate.

The baccalaureate degree program in nursing, offered by an institution of higher education, provides learners with the opportunity to acquire knowledge of the theories and practices of nursing; competency in selecting, synthesizing, and applying relevant learnings from other disciplines and fields; the ability to assess nursing needs and to provide nursing intervention; and the ability to evaluate current practices and try new approaches. A leader must have a complete and thorough knowledge of the discipline and the work to be performed before attempting to lead others. A nurse leader is unable to function merely with applied or "how-to-do-it" knowledge. One who has acquired how-to-do knowledge with a minimum amount of theory, defined as the knowledge of the nature, purpose, structure, and function of "what it is" that must be accomplished, is a technician.[42] A technician may be and usually is a very skilled worker, but certainly not a professional or a leader. A technician lacks knowledge of what and why he is doing whatever is being done at every stage of the work. Technicians apply the knowledge and theories created and developed by others. Only a professional nurse with a baccalaureate degree in nursing has acquired a body of theoretical knowledge of nursing as well as applied knowledge. Professional nurses with appropriate theoretical knowledge implement theories of nursing, improvise, and create new nursing techniques within the field based on newly acquired knowledge.

The leadership process in nursing may only be implemented completely, effectively, and expeditiously by persons who have mastered the theoretical knowledge needed to engage in the practice of nursing. A nurse leader must systematically apply nursing knowledge in concrete situations, with persons, families, and in communities, and be able to construct new nursing theories where required.

The characteristics of graduate education in nursing include in-depth specialization in an area of interest, mastery of nursing knowledge, inquiry and pursuit of more and new knowledge, the acquisition of new skills, and the competence in research to develop and build nursing knowledge. A distinction may be made that baccalaureate nursing graduates are prepared for leadership in nursing with persons, families, and communities. Masters and higher degree nurse graduates are prepared for leadership beyond and within the total health care delivery systems, in a specialized way, in all institutes of nursing at the national and international level.

The stated premises and the nursing leadership process lend themselves to verification by research within the nursing setting.

It must be pointed out that a successful leader is one who facilitates the determination and achievement of desirable goals, consistent with characteristics and cultural expectations of the present day. The style of leadership accommodates the demands of the situation and is determined by the composition of behaviors incorporated in the nursing leadership process utilized by the leader. Since nursing situations are complex, having many variables inherent in the situation—crisis situations, well situations—so that thinking time may be short, moderate, or involve a long time, the nursing leader must have mastered the leadership process behaviors to accommodate a changing scene. Any one nurse leader will encounter, in any one day, situations demanding a large range of behaviors. No effort will be spent on describing leadership styles, which are readily available in the literature. The value of nursing leadership behaviors rests with a group of persons in a particular situation at a given time. The focus must be on the dimensions of nursing leadership behavior implied in the nursing leadership process utilized in a changing, fluctuating, human situation requiring nursing, whenever, with whomever, and wherever it occurs.

To conclude, following a review and selection of the theoretical formulations for leadership deemed most useful for the nursing setting, a definition of leadership and nursing leadership was developed in keeping with and complementary to the definition of leadership developed by Stogdill, based on research results. He defines leadership as the initiation and maintenance of structure in expectation and interaction. He indicates further that the leader plays an active part in developing and maintaining role structure and goal direction, which are strategic for effective role performance.[43]

By defining leadership as the process of influencing the behavior of other persons in their effort toward goal setting and achievement, and nursing leadership as the process whereby a person, who is a nurse, affects the actions of others in goal determination and achievement, the focus was set for the determination of the nursing leadership process, the development of the taxonomy of behaviors relating to the nursing leadership process, and the designation of the dimensions of the process.

Inherent in the definitions used is goal determination, which adds the structure for pursuit of goal achievement. The time and distance from the goal determination to achievement depends on the ability of the leader to decide, relate, influence, and facilitate the action(s) of the followers. This focus is on the here and now but proceeds into the future. Goal determination remains an idea until it becomes operationalized, either in the present or in the future. The span of activity to meet the goals may be short, intermediate, and long range.

The style of nursing leadership and the effectiveness of nursing leadership are inherent in the leader's demonstration of behaviors related to each component of the nursing leadership process.

The logical next step to the determination of the nursing leadership process is the education of persons who can utilize this process.

References

1. Stogdill R: Handbook of Leadership. New York, Free Press, 1974.
2. Leadership. Edited by CA Gibbs. Baltimore, Penguin Books, 1969, p 201.
3. Tannenbaum R, Weschler I, Massarik F: Leadership and Organization. New York, McGraw-Hill Book Co, 1961, p 24.
4. *Idem:* p 26.
5. *Idem:* p 26.
6. *Idem:* pp 28-29.
7. *Idem:* p 28.
8. *Idem:* p 31.
9. *Idem:* pp 31-42.
10. *Idem:* p 34.
11. Stogdill R: Individual Behavior and Group Achievement. New York, Oxford Press, 1959, p 12.
12. *Idem:* pp 12-14.

13. *Idem:* p 21.
14. *Idem:* pp 40-41.
15. *Idem:* p 63.
16. *Idem:* pp 72-73.
17. *Idem:* p 82.
18. *Idem:* p 122.
19. *Idem:* pp 122-123.
20. *Idem:* p 285.
21. *Idem:* p 201.
22. Griffiths D: Administrative Theory. New York, Appleton-Century-Crofts, 1959, p 75.
23. *Idem:* p 94.
24. Gibbs CA: The principles and traits of leadership, Leadership. Edited by CA Gibbs. Baltimore, Penguin Books, 1969, pp 211-212.
25. Fiedler F: A Theory of Leadership Effectiveness. New York, McGraw-Hill Book Co., 1967, pp 5-6.
26. Stogdill R: Handbook of Leadership. New York, Free Press, 1974, p 65.
27. *Idem:* p 81.
28. *Idem:* p 344.
29. *Idem:* p 344.
30. *Idem:* p 231.
31. *Idem:* p 96.
32. Barnard C: The Functions of the Executive. Cambridge, Harvard University Press, 1964, p 108.
33. Jay A: Corporation Man. New York, Random House, 1971, p 19.
34. *Idem:* p 20.
35. *Idem:* p 33.
36. *Idem:* p 51.
37. Webster's New World Dictionary of the American Language. New York, World Publishing Co, 1960, pp 19, 890, 1465.
38. Webster's New Twentieth Century Dictionary of the English Language, unabridged. New York, Standard Reference Works Publishing Company, 1956, pp 24, 972, 1028, 1713.
39. Jay A: Corporation Man. New York, Random House, 1971, p 67.
40. Aikens C: Hospital Training-School Methods and the Head Nurse. Philadelphia, WB Saunders Co, 1914, p 18
41. Yura, H, Walsh M: The Nursing Process. New York, Appleton-Century-Crofts, 1973, p 20.
42. Hanlon J: Theory and the practice of nursing. J Cont Ed Nurs 5:15, Nov-Dec 1974.
43. Stogdill R: Handbook of Leadership. New York, Free Press, 1974, p 411.

CHAPTER 4
Educational Preparation for Nursing Leadership Development

The only way to ensure that nursing will have the leaders it needs is to prepare them deliberately. Expecting leaders to develop spontaneously or to emerge automatically is unrealistic. It is unlikely that such a "hit-or-miss" method would resolve nursing's leadership dilemma. Rather, it would contribute to it.

The expectations and mechanisms for the preparation of nurse leaders already exist in nursing. Graduates of baccalaureate and masters degree programs in nursing are expected to be leaders. However, this expectation, although clear, does not ensure that leaders will be prepared. A well-thought-out description of the behavioral expectations for the development of nursing leadership for each step in the academic preparation of nurses at the baccalaureate and masters degree levels must be determined. Following this, the specific learning—both theoretical and laboratory—needs to be designated to ensure that level behaviors are achieved.

The need deliberately to prepare required leaders has long been encouraged by researchers, authors, and thoughtful citizens across the country. There seems to be strong evidence that a demonstration of leadership behavior in high school and college tends to predict leadership in adult life. Also, there is strong evidence to support the concept that leadership is transferable from one situation to another.[1]

Gardner states that one of the gravest deficiencies is not doing what should be done to encourage potential leaders. There is no reason to doubt that human material is still there, but there is strong support for the belief that it is either not being developed or is being diverted into nonleadership activities.[2] He further points out that "we educate the technical expert who advises the leader, but no one will want to educate the leader himself."[3] "Nursing also has lagged remarkably in failing to encourage the development of sufficient numbers of able leaders. Hope for the future lies in those who are privileged to partake of higher learning and more particularly in those who are recognized for their leadership abilities."[4]

Nursing must plan for and develop leaders by deliberately selecting persons who can be encouraged to develop their minds and to acquire sufficient nursing knowledge and wisdom so that their colleagues grant them the privilege of charting the course of the profession of nursing.[5] Special effort should be made to identify these intellectually oriented, capable students early in their college careers, preferably in the freshman year. Then specific arrangements should be made to involve them in the academic life of the university and to support and nurture them in their professionalization as well as to develop their leadership potential. It may be necessary to design individually tailored programs and to provide guidance services to help maintain interest, a willingness to serve, and a desire to pursue a leadership role.[6]

A major task of nursing leaders today is the identification and development of nurse leaders who will vitalize society and a significant component of this society—nursing.

> Nursing has far too long been guilty of promoting conformists and of being punitive to those who are innovative and creative. The field suffers from a dearth of persons whose motivations and discoveries have vitalized the profession. . . . The demonstration of real leadership in nursing will come when those who are now leaders in the

Educational Preparation for Nursing Leadership Development 135

field identify, foster, and promote the deliberate preparation of their successors.[7]

Although there is no shortage of admonitions that persons with leadership potential must be identified first, and then deliberately and carefully developed, little has been accomplished in a practical sense.

In 1969 a descriptive survey was done of faculty perceptions of behavior indicating leadership potential of baccalaureate nursing students. The leader-behavior categories identified related to knowledge of self, critical thinking, interpersonal relationships, and group and job relations. These were supported by the respondents.[8] Unless the nursing leadership process, which can be learned and nurtured, is specified, little definitive success would be realized by those who are to prepare the leaders. In addition to learning to decide, relate, influence, and facilitate, other expectations include acquiring and retaining the leadership role, maintaining this role even when its legitimacy is obviously challenged, demonstrating leadership behavior in varied nursing situations, sensitivity and analysis of the effects of leadership behavior on group performance and on member satisfaction, and continuing research in nursing leadership, particularly the nursing leadership process.[9]

In an effort to determine whether the nursing faculty had explicated a nursing leadership process and whether nurse leaders were deliberately prepared in baccalaureate and masters degree programs in nursing, an extensive review of self-evaluation reports was undertaken. The total sample of available reports ($N = 248$), based on the 1969 and 1972 *Criteria for the Appraisal of Baccalaureate and Higher Degree Programs in Nursing,* for presentation to the Board of Review for Baccalaureate and Higher Degree Programs and available for research and for faculty study were reviewed.[10] Evidence for any and all statements relating to leadership was sought throughout the self-study reports.

In the philosophies of programs under review statements were readily found that tended to be beliefs that students in baccalaureate and masters degree programs were being prepared to assume leadership roles in nursing. Following through on these beliefs by seeking evidence in curricular materials to show that they were being implemented produced disappointing revelations. Although a few self-studies included definitions of leadership and/or descriptions of the content of courses, such as leadership theory, little other than a statement of philosophy of leadership could be found. It was rare to find a deliberate determination of terminal, level, and course behaviors that could result in the development of leadership behaviors. In only one instance was there reference to a leadership process. Frequently, a course entitled "leadership in nursing" was offered in the second semester of the senior year. Further inspection revealed that this was a course in team leading in an acute care setting. Courses in management could be found more often. It is particularly important to note that little could be found on the nursing care of groups of individuals and families except in the acute care setting. If considerations were given to long-term, home care, and well settings, these were not included in course materials. More often, as noted earlier, courses were offered in team leadership or management in nursing. Only in a few reports was there some evidence of a logical, sequential attempt to provide theory and laboratory experiences for leadership development.

The leadership references were rare in the review of reports on masters programs in nursing. This was a direct contrast to what was expected. Although references were found in programs in which a philosophy of leadership was stated, these were generally the only ones in the report. In a few programs offering courses of study in nursing education and nursing service administration, the focus was on administration and management theory and administration and management process, with some reference to leadership. In programs that excluded administration as a course of study and in which clinical specialization was emphasized, theoretical and laboratory experiences specifically directed toward leadership development were almost nonexistent. References to leadership were found when the preparation of administrators was the aim, in contrast to the preparation of specialist nursing practitioners, researchers, consultants, and teachers.

It was rare to find reference to the contribution of general education to the preparation of nurse leaders, ie, the biologic, physical, social, and behavioral sciences that form the basis for courses required for professional nursing majors or which are taught concurrently with that major.

To conclude, little information was found in the review of self-study reports that clearly outlined the deliberate preparation of nurse leaders. When references were found, they were usually in the curricular materials available for the baccalaureate degree program in nursing. Although students were exposed to a variety of general and liberal educational material, there was no evidence to indicate that these contributed to the preparation of the nurse leader. In a few instances, the term *change agent* was used as a synonym for leader. However, in some reports the terms *nurse leader* and *change agent* were used interchangeably. There was no indication that change theory and the change process were part of the curriculum.

It is important to note that in the accreditation process no criterion relating to leadership development was a part of the *Criteria for the Appraisal of Baccalaureate and Higher Degree Programs* until 1972. This criterion requires that "both theory and practice provide for the development of leadership skills."[10] This may account in part for the lack of references to leadership in studies based on the 1969 criteria and the somewhat more obvious statements in those self-study reports based on the 1972 criteria. However, this alone does not account for the fact that in stated philosophies for the program in which the terms *nurse leader* or *change agent* appeared, clearly defined sequential learnings were not found that would assure formal preparation of nurse leaders.

Although it is true that any nurse who uses all four components in the nursing leadership process is deemed a leader, the formal deliberate preparation of this leader is the task of the baccalaureate and masters degree programs in nursing. It is these programs at colleges and universities across the country that will prepare the nurse leader to lead and relate to a diverse public—clients, colleagues, co-professionals, such as physicians, dentists, clergy, lawyers, as well as community, political, and educational leaders. The number of different public groups with whom nurse leaders deal, as well as the number of relationships between and among the groups, strains the nurse leader's ability to decide, relate, influence, and facilitate interchange to a far greater extent than for leaders in other areas or with one or a limited number of public groups. The nurse's role is one of the most difficult in society; therefore the nursing leadership role is one of the most demanding.

To be adequately prepared for their roles, nurse leaders require a broad background of knowledge related to man, society, health, and nursing, as well as specific knowledge on which to base decisions and on how to relate, influence, and facilitate. An analysis of what the nurse leader needs to know and do is given below. It should be noted that some of what the nurse leader is required to learn is needed to utilize the nursing and research processes. The list of what must be learned is divided among the categories deciding, relating, influencing, and facilitating. Each of these categories of learning requisites contains studies relating to man, society, health, and nursing.

DECIDING

Knowledge Delineation

What knowledge the nurse leader must have:
- Society, its structure, participants, needs, and goals
- Social, political, and health issues confronting society, generally, and the United States of America, specifically
- Behavior—individual, family, and community
- Environmental determinants affecting human endeavors
- Social, political, and health issues confronting nursing
- Standards of living—local, state, regional, national, and international
- Health organization and health resources
- Present health service delivery system in the United States of America
- Economics of health and illness
- Legal aspects of health care and nursing practice
- Communication within formal and informal organizations
- Policy development
- Roles and relations of broad range of health service personnel
- Role of and functional differences between vocational, technical, professional generalist, and professional specialist nursing practitioners
- Opinions, stereotypes, and expectations of citizens regarding health and nursing service personnel

Significant historic dimensions of nursing
Standards of practice—nursing and medical
Nursing theory (theories)
Nursing process
Research process
The future direction of nursing
Impact of self on others
Systems theory
Decision theory
Change theory
Need theory
The scientific method
Distinction between problem solving and the scientific method
Application of the scientific method
Statistical methods
How to identify a problem
How to hypothesize
How to assess a situation
What constitutes a data base
Sources of information
How to collect data, from whom, and from where
How to discriminate between fact, fiction, opinion, principles, law, and theory
How to discriminate between and among data
How to predict the consequences of action
How to validate inferences
Reporting and recording data and decisions
Auditing procedures and practices
Multiple influences on thinking, including cultural, ethnic, racial, religious, territorial, socioeconomic, and age dimensions
The influence of stress on thinking
Deviant thinking patterns

Behavioral Counterparts

What the nurse leader can do:
  Utilize knowledge of society, its structure, participants, needs, and goals for consumer and nursing purposes
  Demonstrate a working knowledge of social, political, and health

issues confronting society, partciularly the United States of America

Utilize a knowledge of behavior in dealing with individuals, families, and communities

Be sensitive to the environmental determinants affecting human endeavors

Determine, evaluate, and affect the social, political, and health issues confronting nursing

Operationalize research results relating to men, society, health, and nursing in meeting the goals of nursing

Incorporate knowledge of standards of living on the local, state, regional, national, and international levels in affecting change to enhance the health status of the citizens

Demonstrate a working knowledge of the present national health service delivery system

Demonstrate an appreciation of the economics of health and illness on the individual, the family, the community, and the nation

Practice within the legal framework for health care and nursing care

Demonstrate a working knowledge of the system of communication within formal and informal organizations

Demonstrate a working knowledge of policy development within the formal and informal organization

Distinguish the roles and relations of the broad range of health service personnel

Distinguish the role and functional differences of vocational, technical, professional generalist nursing practitioner and professional specialist nursing practitioner, including the complementary aspects of these roles and functions

Demonstrate an awareness of opinions, stereotypes, and expectations of citizens regarding health and nursing service personnel with plans to correct distortions

Determine the significant historic dimensions of nursing and their influence on present and future directions in nursing

Utilize present standards for nursing and medical practice as a basis for comparison and change

Demonstrate a knowledge of prevailing nursing theories as well as one's own theory of nursing

Demonstrate mastery of the nursing process

Utilize the research process in the nursing situation

Influence the future direction of nursing

Demonstrate sensitivity to the impact of self on others

Utilize systems theory in nursing practice

Utilize decision theory in nursing practice
Utilize change theory in influencing and determining the direction of change in individuals and groups
Demonstrate the use of need theory in determining needs of self, individuals, groups, and communities
Utilize the scientific method to test hypotheses relating to nursing practice
Readily distinguish the difference between problem solving and the scientific method in nursing practice
Apply the scientific method in nursing practice
Utilize statistical methods and interpret results of this utilization
Identify a problem, determine strategies to resolve the problem, then implement and evaluate the strategy
Hypothesize about problems related to nursing practice
Test hypotheses and determine the results and applicability of results
Assess a situation
Determine the components of the situation
Designate if a plan of action would be needed
Utilize sources of information from multiple sources simultaneously
Demonstrate data collection from a variety of sources—persons, records—wherever data are found
Discriminate between fact, fiction, opinion, principles, laws, and theory
Discriminate data
Predict consequences of action
Validate inferences
Record and report data and decisions
Demonstrate knowledge of auditing procedures and practices
Demonstrate knowledge of multiple influences on thinking, including cultural, ethnic, racial, religious, territorial, socioeconomic, and age dimensions
Demonstrate knowledge of the influence of stress on thinking
Diagnose deviant thinking patterns

RELATING

Knowledge Delineation

What knowledge the nurse leader must have:
Human behavior
Basic human needs

Human growth and development
Mental mechanisms
Deviant behavior
How to foster behavioral change
How to develop self
Influence of self on others
Self-evaluation
Self-reflection
The learning process
The teaching process
Multiple techniques to facilitate learning for self and others
Group behavior and process
Group norms and group growth patterns
Influence of individuals on group and group on individuals
Methods of individual and group goal determination
Family
How to assess individual and family coping ability
Role theory
Religions, ethical, ethnic, cultural, racial, and socioeconomic influences on human behavior—individual, group, and community
Mechanism of change on individual, group, and community
How to relate to others
Communication theory
Use of language
Language, symbols, and meaning
Use of symbols in communicating
Verbal and nonverbal communication
Physical dimensions in relating and communicating
Cultural influences in relating and communicating
Educational influences in relating and communicating
Social influences in relating and communicating
Masculine and feminine influences in relating and communicating
Psychologic influences in relating and communicating
Influence of age in relating and communicating
Geographic and climatic influences in relating and communicating
Dimensions of touch in relating and communicating
Silence in relating and communicating
Influence of listening in relating and communicating
Environmental influences on individual and group behavior
Territoriality and personal space as they influence relating and communicating

Dimensions of confidentiality and privacy in relating and communicating
Ethical and moral dimensions of relating and communicating
How to extract meaning from communication
Communication techniques as questioning, reflecting, and others
Interviewing
How to elicit information
What constitutes needed health information
How to initiate a relationship
How to continue a relationship
How and when to terminate a relationship

Behavioral Counterparts

What the nurse leader can do:
Utilize a knowledge of human behavior in relating with clients, colleagues, and co-workers
Demonstrate a mastery of basic human needs as the territory for nursing practice
Demonstrate a working knowledge of human growth and development
Determine the use of and the meaning of mental mechanisms
Distinguish between normal and deviant human behavior
Determine the direction and mechanism of needed behavioral change
Focus on the continuing development of the self
Be sensitive to the influence of self on others
Evaluate self in relation to stated expectations and objectives
Reflect upon self as a means of self-improvement and enhancing self-awareness
Demonstrate a mastery of the learning process as applied to self and others
Demonstrate mastery of the teaching process in relation to clients, colleagues, students, and co-workers
Utilize multiple techniques selectively to facilitate learning for self and others
Determine group behavior and the operational group process
Account for group norms and group growth patterns in actual nursing situations
Demonstrate an awareness of the influence of the individual on the group and the group on the individual
Be sensitive to the manner and methods of goal determination by individuals and groups

Draw upon a knowledge of the family to enhance relating with the family

Assess individual and family coping ability as it relates to health

Utilize the knowledge of role theory in determining, establishing, and understanding roles and relationships of individuals and groups in the nursing situation

Demonstrate a working knowledge of the religious, ethical, ethnic, cultural, racial, and socioeconomic influences of the behavior of the individuals, groups, and communities comprising the leader's public

Demonstrate an awareness of how changes occur and how these changes influence the individual, the group, and the community

Relate easily and effectively with others

Operationalize knowledge of communication theory

Demonstrate mastery in the use of language including the influences as culturally, socially, ethnically, racially, and economically determined

Demonstrate an appreciation of language, symbols, and the inherent meanings

Demonstrate mastery in the utilization and determination of verbal and nonverbal communication

Be considerate of the physical dimensions of relating and communicating

Be aware of the educational influences in relating and communicating

Determine the social influences in relating and communicating

Account for the masculine and feminine influences in relating and communicating

Determine the psychologic influences in relating and communicating

Be sensitive to the influence of age and age differences in relating and communicating

Determine the geographic and climatic influences in relating and communicating

Appreciate the dimensions of touch in relating and communicating with determination of its uses

Determine the use and impact of silence in relating and communicating

Determine when listening should prevail in relating and communicating

Determine the influence of environment on individual and group behavior

Determine the influence of territoriality and personal space as they influence relating and communicating

Maintain appropriate confidentiality and privacy in relating and communicating

Demonstrate ethical and moral dimensions in relating and communicating
Extract meaning from communication
Utilize, appropriately, communication techniques such as questioning, reflecting, and others
Interview
Elicit information
Demonstrate a knowledge of what constitutes needed health information
Initiate, continue, and terminate a relationship

INFLUENCING

Knowledge Delineation

What knowledge the nurse leader must have:
  Societal forces and constraints
  Social organization
  Communities, their purposes, and composition
  Political organization and influences
  Political process in formal and informal organization, in local, state, regional, national, and international circles
  Power and the holders of power—individuals, groups, communities, nations, and the world
  Power structures in nursing
  Historic perspectives of nursing
  Prominent persons in legislative, health, education, industry, government, and nursing circles
  Legal processes
  Broad range of possible goals for human endeavor
  Consumer needs for health and nursing service
  Health organizations
  Stages of human development
  Basic human needs
  Individual needs and differences
  Personality development
  Population, division of labor, and roles in society
  Cultural dimensions and impact on person, group, and community
  Role theory

Stress theory
Crisis theory
Change process
Self
Use of self
How to express self clearly and logically
Behavioral adaptation to changing situations
Group process
How individuals and groups determine goals
Ways to modify behavior
The world of work
Needs met by work
Effect of rewards and punishment (withholding of reward) on individual and group behavior
Human response to reward and punishment
Individual performance needs and differences
How to support purposeful human efforts
Ways people communicate with each other
Methods of human confrontation
How to withdraw from a relationship or how to prevent a relationship from developing
Human response to pressure and stress
Effect of stress on thinking
How to appeal to individuals and groups
Formal and informal organizations
How to transact
How to requisition
How to allocate
Budgeting
How to give instructions
How to negotiate and bargain
How to delegate
Methods to convey information and awareness of societal issues
Mass media methodologies
Audiovisual techniques
Advertising process
How to think critically
How to judge the relevance of data
How to deliberate about data
How to make a nursing judgment

Educational Preparation for Nursing Leadership Development 147

    Range of choices available to solve a problem
    Broad range of strategies to accomplish a task
    How to determine goals
    What constitutes a risk
    How to set priorities
    How to plan
    How to designate modes of action to achieve goals
    How to influence the views and actions of others
    How to put a plan into operation
    How to modify action to fit the situation
    How to evaluate performance of self
    How to evaluate performance of co-workers and colleagues
    Motivation—its development and impact
    How to write and publish information, ideas, rationales, and strategies
    Accountability and morality in deciding, relating, influencing, and facilitating

INFLUENCING

Behavioral Counterparts

What the nurse leader can do:
    Demonstrate a knowledge of societal forces and constraints as a basis for the determination of planned action
    Determine and describe social organization
    Determine the purposes and composition of communities where nursing practice occurs
    Demonstrate a working knowledge of the political process in formal and informal organizations and in local, state, regional, national, and international circles
    Demonstrate a grasp of the power structure and power holders whether among individuals, groups, communities, nations, and the world
    Determine the power structures in nursing
    Demonstrate an historic perspective of nursing
    Relate to prominent persons in legislative, health, educational, industrial, governmental, and nursing circles
    Demonstrate grasp of the legal process
    Demonstrate a broad range of possible goals for human endeavor
    Determine consumer needs for health and nursing service

Explain the prevailing patterns of health organization
Assess the stages of human development
Determine the status of fulfillment of basic human needs
Appreciate individual needs and differences
Demonstrate a working knowledge of personality development
Utilize knowledge of population, division of labor, and roles in determining nursing actions
Designate the cultural dimensions and their impact on the person, group, and community
Operationalize knowledge of role theory in the nursing setting
Operationalize knowledge of stress theory in the nursing situation
Operationalize knowledge of crisis theory in the nursing situation
Demonstrate use of the change process
Demonstrate an appreciation and knowledge of self
Demonstrate use of self
Express self clearly and logically
Adapt behavior to changing situations
Utilize knowledge of group process
Support the efforts of individuals and groups in goal determination
Effectively modify behavior of self and others
Demonstrate grasp of the world of work for self and others
Demonstrate awareness of the needs met by engagement in work
Demonstrate a knowledge of the effect of reward and punishment on individual and group behavior
Demonstrate an appreciation of the human response of individuals to the use of reward and punishment
Determine individual performance needs and differences
Demonstrate support of purposeful human effort
Demonstrate mastery of the ways people communicate with each other
Demonstrate a working knowledge of methods of human confrontation
Determine how and when to withdraw from a relationship and how to prevent a relationship from developing
Be sensitive to human response to pressure and stress
Determine the effect of stress on thinking
Appeal to individuals and groups in goal designation
Demonstrate a working knowledge of formal and informal organization
Transact business
Requisition needed resources—persons, money, facilities, and supplies
Demonstrate the ability to allocate money, services, and supplies
Prepare a budget

Give instructions to clients, coworkers, and colleagues
Negotiate and bargain for needed human and monetary resources
Delegate action to be accomplished by selected knowledgeable persons
Convey information about and awareness of societal issues affecting nursing education and nursing service
Utilize mass media methodologies
Demonstrate audiovisual techniques
Demonstrate knowledge and use of advertising process
Determine appropriate promotional techniques
Demonstrate mastery in the use of the problem-solving process
Demonstrate ability to think critically
Judge the relevance of data
Deliberate about data
Make a nursing judgment
Select from a range of choices the strategy or strategies appropriate to accomplish a task
Determine goals for self and with other persons and groups
Analyze the extent of risk taking
Set priorities
Plan for self, with, and for others—clients, co-workers, and colleagues
Designate modes of action to achieve goals
Influence the views and actions of clients, co-workers, and colleagues
Put a plan into operation
Modify action to fit the situation
Evaluate performance of self
Evaluate performance of co-workers and colleagues
Demonstrate a knowledge of motivation, its development and its impact
Write and publish information, ideas, rationales, and strategies
Demonstrate accountability and morality in deciding, relating, influencing, and facilitating

FACILITATING

Knowledge Delineation

What knowledge the nurse leader must have:
Epidemiology
Statistical methods
Resources relating to man, health, society, and nursing

Media and library resources, including major indexes, references, services, and others
Aspiration of individuals and groups from a broad range of national, cultural, ethnic, and geographic areas
Broad range of resources—human, group, community, national, and international
Finance
Economic resources
How to deal with economic resources
Communication patterns in official, nonofficial, governmental, nongovernmental, temporary, and permanent human organizations
How to intervene to improve varied processes—communication, group, nursing, research
How to initiate contacts with influential individuals and groups
The impact of control as a dimension in individual, group, and organizational behavior
Historic dimension of goal achievement
Authority structure in formal and informal organizations
Power structure in formal and informal organizations
Committee organization
Patterns of relating to other persons in an organizational structure
Administrative, management, and supervisory processes
Functional roles of individual and group members in informal and formal organizations
How persons behave in their roles
Personnel needs
Need for personnel to accomplish a task
How to foster a helping relationship
Intergroup relations
Interpersonal relations
Dimensions of interdisciplinary education and practice
Problem prevention
Communication patterns in formal and informal organizations
Risks involved in planned action
How to delegate
How to coordinate
How to realize goal achievement
Alternative patterns of action to achieve a specified goal
How to initiate and direct change
How to maintain continued human effort throughout the change process

How to compromise
Work flow
Production
Budgetary responsibility
Coping mechanisms
Principles of learning and teaching
Teaching strategies
When, where, how and with whom the facilitating of interaction and action occurs
How to develop needed resources

Behavioral Counterparts

What the nurse leader can do:
  Demonstrate a working knowledge of epidemiologic content
  Use a variety of statistical methods, including ability to interpret results
  Demonstrate a working knowledge of the major resources relating to man, health, society, and nursing
  Utilize media and library resources including major indexes, references, and services as a means of facilitating action
  Be sensitive to the aspirations of individuals and groups from a broad range of national, cultural, ethnic, and geographic areas when facilitating the purposeful actions of individuals and groups
  Demonstrate mastery of a broad range of resources—human, group, community, national, and international
  Demonstrate a working knowledge of finance
  Demonstrate ability to deal with economic resources
  Determine communication patterns in official, nonofficial, governmental, nongovernmental, temporary, and permanent human organizations
  Intervene to improve various processes strategic to nursing practice—communication, group, nursing, and research
  Initiate contacts with influential individuals and groups
  Be sensitive to the impact of control as a dimension in individual, group, and organizational behavior
  Trace historic dimension of goal achievement
  Determine authority structure in formal and informal organization
  Determine power structure in formal and informal organizations
  Demonstrate a working knowledge of committee organization, purposes, and structure

Determine patterns of relating and communicating with persons in an organizational structure

Determine and distinguish between the administrative, management, and supervisory processes

Determine functional roles of individual and group members in informal and formal organizations

Determine how persons behave in their personal, family, and occupational roles

Designate need for personnel considering the qualifications, competencies, and numbers needed

Be sensitive to the need for personnel to accomplish a task

Foster a helping relationship with clients, colleagues, and co-workers

Demonstrate awareness of the range and impact of intergroup relations

Demonstrate knowledge of human relations in day-to-day human endeavors

Demonstrate awareness of the dimensions of interdisciplinary education and practice

Demonstrate sensitivity to opportunities for problem prevention

Determine communication patterns in formal and informal organizations

Determine and take risks involved in planned action

Delegate appropriately and effectively

Coordinate actions of groups of persons—clients, colleagues, and co-workers

Demonstrate ability to foster goal achievement

Determine from a range of patterns of actions those most likely to facilitate the achievement of a specified goal

Initiate and direct change

Maintain continued human effort throughout the change process

Compromise with others and promote compromise among relating individuals and groups

Determine work flow

Determine amount, level of, and structure for production

Demonstrate budgetary responsibility

Be sensitive to a range of coping mechanisms employed by individuals, families, and groups

Demonstrate use of the principles of learning and teaching

Demonstrate competence in utilization of teaching strategies

Demonstrate when, where, how, and for whom facilitating interaction and action occurs

Develop resources as needed to facilitate action

The range of knowledge and behavioral counterparts presented should be continuously elaborated upon by nurse educators. No attempt was made to discriminate between those appropriate to the baccalaureate or masters degree programs in nursing. The nursing faculty for these programs must determine what the nursing student is required to know, the depth of such knowledge, and in which programs (total curriculum and specific courses) the required learnings are to be included.

If the nursing faculty has expressed its belief that the leader is prepared in the baccalaureate and masters degree programs in nursing, then this belief should be carried to fruition. In other words, the curriculum should include evidence that the leader in nursing is being prepared and will be fully capable of assuming that role in practice.

BACCALAUREATE NURSING EDUCATION

The baccalaureate degree program in nursing is designed to prepare the generalist nursing practitioner. Its objectives are to provide the student with a general knowledge of the biologic, physical, social, and behavioral sciences upon which the nursing major is based and from which the rationale for nursing action is drawn. Another objective describes the nursing process as the core process for the practice of nursing with application to persons and families who are well or ill in whatever setting they are found, incorporating appropriate research findings to the nursing service rendered. Still another objective of the baccalaureate degree program is to prepare a nursing leader who can coordinate efforts for consumer health and nursing service, act as a colleague in concert with other health professionals, encourage change in the quality and direction of health and nursing services, and at the same time foster one's own personal and professional growth. A final objective is to offer a base for the pursuit of graduate education in nursing.

To put these objectives into operation, clearly stated behavioral expectations for the graduate of the baccalaureate degree program are needed. The behavioral expectations flow directly from the objectives and when completed provide a profile of the graduate of the program. In other words, the behavioral statements describe the graduate in terms of what she knows and can do.

The focus in the baccalaureate degree program in nursing is greatest in the direction of intellectual skills, such as problem solving, deciding, thinking critically, and making nursing judgments. Interpersonal skills, such as relating, interviewing, information gathering, providing information, conveying interest, concern, and compassion, as well as data-gathering and interventive skills of a technical nature are learned.

Baccalaureate graduates in nursing are prepared for a high degree of independent and interdependent practice, with limited, reasoned, dependent aspects. Even these limited dependent aspects of practice are viewed by some as independent and interdependent because of the high level of intellectual input needed to judge the appropriate and legal limit of participation.

In November 1974 the Council of Baccalaureate and Higher Degree Programs voted to accept the proposed Characteristics of Baccalaureate Education in Nursing. Clearly stated within this document is the notion that students in the baccalaureate degree program in nursing should have an opportunity to acquire knowledge of the developing theories and practices of nursing; knowledge of the broad function the profession is expected to perform in society; competency in selecting, synthesizing, and applying relevant information from various disciplines; competency in collaborating with members of other disciplines and with consumers; the ability to assess nursing needs and provide nursing intervention; the ability to evaluate current practices and try new approaches; and a foundation for graduate study in nursing.[11] More specifically, the Council membership determined that graduates of the baccalaureate degree program in nursing were able to (a) utilize theoretical and empirical knowledge from the physical and behavioral sciences and the humanities as a source of making nursing practice decisions; (b) utilize the nursing process in that the graduate could assess health status and health potential, plan, implement, and evaluate nursing care in concert with clients who are persons, families, or communities. Further, ability to use the nursing process requires the utilization of decision-making theories in determining care plans, designs, or interventions for achieving comprehensive nursing goals. In addition, nursing interventions (part of the planning and implementation phases of the nursing process) are to be utilized as hypotheses to be tested, anticipating a variety of consequences, making predictions, and selecting and evaluating the effectiveness of alternative approaches; (c) accept individual responsibility and accountability for nursing interventions and their results; (d) use nursing practice as a means for gathering data for refining and extending nursing science; (e) share in the responsibility for the health and welfare of all people with citizens and colleagues on the interdisciplinary health team by collaborating, coordinating, and consulting with them; (f) assist in implementing change to improve delivery of health care; and (g) understand present and emerging roles of the professional nurse.[11]

The document further states that the graduate of the baccalaureate degree program in nursing can progress toward acceptance of a greater share of responsibility in the provision of health care services, toward development of more productive methods of working interdependently with other health care professionals, toward realizing a broadened scope of practice, toward greater independence as practitioners, toward acceptance of the advocacy role in relation to clients and toward promoting the self-understanding, the personal fulfillment, and the motivation for continual learning to maintain expertise in the area of nursing practice.

In this atmosphere, and within the community of scholars, leaders for nursing are prepared to guarantee that behavioral expectations for the prescribed graduate of the baccalaureate degree program in nursing will be achieved. Other dimensions are needed to complete the curriculum framework. A conceptual framework that must be stated is the designation of significant concepts that flow from philosophy with the designation of theoretical formulations with hypotheses, that describe the concepts, assist in determining the focus and selecting content, and provide the base for ensuing decisions with respect to the curriculum. Significant concepts identified by nursing faculty across the country, at this time, are man, society, health, and nursing.[12] Subconcepts for nursing are generally held to be the nursing leadership and research processes.

Once the conceptual framework has been delineated, the next step is to determine the threads or strands that flow from described components of the curricular framework (particularly from the conceptual framework) as they permeate the curriculum. Then the level behavioral expectations are stated. Level behaviors are more specifically stated than are broader behavioral expectations for the program, but level behaviors flow directly from them and account for the conceptual framework and identified threads or strands for each level to be pursued by the prospective student. The level behaviors serve as guideposts along the way to ensure that learnings are logical, sequential, and will operationalize the end of program expectations and, at the same time, meet the objectives for the program.

When level behavioral expectations have been precisely stated, the course behaviors, which flow from these statements of level behavior, are developed. They are stated more specifically than are the level behaviors and include the learnings to be achieved in a course conducted over a short span of time—usually a semester, trimester, or quarter. Course content needed to operationalize the course behavioral expectations must be determined. The content focus in nursing courses should be nursing. The teaching–learning strategies designated to implement, expand, and operationalize the content are selected.

Only in relation to level and course behavioral expectations can the knowledge and behavioral counterparts for the development of the nursing leadership process be cited. The nursing leadership process behavioral statements may comprise behavioral statements or substatements for levels, courses, and specific lesson plans in conjunction with courses. Content and teaching–learning strategies are then developed to ensure that these behavioral expectations are met.

Learnings related to the nursing leadership process begin with the biologic, physical, social, and behavioral sciences which comprise the lower division courses for the professional nursing major and which are continued throughout the program of studies. These learnings are built upon, transferred, expanded, and put into practice in the nursing courses. A systematic plan to evaluate the curricular framework, the total, its parts, and its participants (students, faculty, as well as graduates of the program) must be developed to ensure that all predetermined behavioral expectations have been achieved by the graduate of the program, including those behaviors related to the nursing leadership process. Actually, the graduate should have mastered the nursing process, the research process, as well as the nursing leadership process. Mastery of this triad of processes comprises the practice of the generalist nursing practitioner.

The first professional degree or the baccalaureate degree program in nursing serves as the base upon which the masters degree program is built.

GRADUATE NURSING EDUCATION

The masters degree program in nursing prepares the specialist nursing practitioner. The specialist builds upon the generalist base already acquired and deepens, extends, and broadens the student's knowledge and skills in the discipline of nursing and concentrates on a particular area of nursing. The graduate of the masters degree program in nursing renders care by focusing on the specific needs of persons and on families with complex health and nursing problems, which specifically designed nursing intervention helps to resolve.[13] This graduate expands and deepens her competency in the triad of processes—nursing, nursing leadership, and research, and implements them in a specialized area. The graduate's high level of ability to decide, relate, influence, and facilitate should come through, no matter what the particular choice for study in nursing or whether the functional areas are clinical specialization, teaching, administration, research, supervision, or consultation. In other words, the academic experience in graduate education in nursing (masters and doctoral level) should build upon and expand the learnings related to the nursing leadership process started at the baccalaureate level in nursing. Whether the graduate functions as a leader in a nursing practice role, as a faculty member, an administrator in nursing education and nursing service, as a researcher, as a consultant, or as a theorist, she is *the* nurse leader wherever and with whomever she functions.

In NLN's Council of Baccalaureate and Higher Degree Program's statement of Characteristics of Graduate Education in Nursing, the general characteristics derived from the purposes of graduate education in nursing are stated to be the preparation of leaders in nursing—those who will influence the practice and study of nursing by generating higher levels of competency and by teaching, administering, and investigating professional practice. It is expected that the graduate student in nursing is a critical, self-directed practitioner, an effective leader in nursing, and a productive contributor to the profession of nursing.[14] More specifically, this graduate develops and tests nursing theories, advances knowledge in the field of nursing through systematic observation and experimentation, relates basic science theories to the development of knowledge in the areas chosen for nursing specialization, identifies and implements nursing's leadership role within the health care delivery system, engages in a collaborative role with others interested in health care, and demonstrates self-understanding, personal fulfillment, and motivation for continued learning.

To ensure that graduate programs in nursing truly build upon and expand the learnings related to the nursing process, the nursing leadership process, and the research process, curricula for the baccalaureate, masters, and doctoral programs in nursing should be developed in concert by responsible nursing faculty. This would be the best insurance that the beliefs inherent in the philosophy are complete, clear, viable, realistic, and supportive of varying levels of practitioner preparation—generalist and specialist.

Accountability for the products of the programs as well as the clear distinctions that exist in terms of the expectations of the graduates can be more readily assured. Although there are distinctions, there are also core elements (the processes of nursing, nursing leadership and research) that have been implanted long before the nursing student takes the first nursing course. Behavioral expectations related to the nursing leadership process need to be carefully delineated and prescribed for each step in the curriculum, on and into graduate educational programs in nursing to ensure that all knowledges and competencies are achieved and that there are no gaps in the preparation of the leader for nursing. Only when the nursing leadership process is taught and then evaluated for learning can nursing be assured of prepared nurse leaders in the numbers needed, rather than hope that leaders will be developed by happenstance.

The only feasible way to ensure a supply of leaders for nursing is by a deliberate effort to prepare leaders, to force those with leadership potential to emerge, to educate for leading by carefully designed learning experiences in which students acquire expertise in deciding, relating, influencing, and facilitating in conjuncton with mastery of the nursing and research processes.

References

1. Stogdill R: The Handbook of Leadership. New York, Free Press, 1974, pp 173-176.
2. Gardner J: The Antileadership Vaccine. Carnegie Corp, New York, Annual Report, New York, 1965, p 9.
3. Gardner J: p 10-11.
4. Schlotfeldt R: Knowledge, leaders, and progress. Image 2:3, 1968.
5. *Idem:* p 2.
6. Kroepsch R: Scaling the academic ranks. Paper presented at meeting of Council of Baccalaureate and Higher Degree Programs in Nursing, National League for Nursing, Cleveland, March 27, 1968, p 8 (Mimeographed).
7. Schlotfeldt R: Knowledge, leaders, and progress. Image 2:5, 1968.
8. Yura H: Faculty Perceptions of behaviors indicating leadership potential of baccalaureate nursing students, unpublished doctoral dissertation, Washington, The Catholic University of America, School of Education, 1970.
9. Stogdill R: The Hankbook of Leadership. New York, Free Press, 1974, p 199.
10. National League for Nursing: Criteria for the Appraisal of Baccalaureate and Higher Degree Programs in Nursing. New York, Council of Baccalaureate and Higher Degree Programs, 1972, p 9.
11. Department of Baccalaureate and Higher Degree Programs: Characteristics of Baccalaureate Education in Nursing. New York, National League for Nursing, 1974.
12. Yura H, Torres G: Conceptual Framework: Its meaning and function. New York, National League for Nursing, 1975.
13. Ozimek D, Yura H: Who is the Nurse Practitioner? New York, National League for Nursing, 1975.
14. Department of Baccalaureate and Higher Degree Programs: Characteristics of Graduate Education in Nursing. New York, National League for Nursing, 1974.

CHAPTER 5
Situational Aspects of Nursing Leadership

In this chapter, two situational aspects for the utilization of the nursing leadership process are presented. The presentations will portray the points of view and functions of two nurse leaders (one from nursing education and one from nursing service) in their specific utilization of the components of the nursing leadership process while simultaneously fostering the use of the process with nursing faculty, students, and staff.

THE NURSING LEADERSHIP PROCESS IN NURSING EDUCATION

Nan Hechenberger

Leadership is a process. It is an abstract rather than a concrete process; it is dynamic rather than static, relative rather than constant, but it is always goal oriented. It is a means to an end, never an end in itself.

Leadership may evolve at any level within an organization. Ideally, it emanates from the top; realistically, it sometimes pushes its way up from the bottom. An administrative position is not essential to the implementation of leadership. In other words, one must be able to exercise leadership if he or she is to succeed as an administrator; however, one does not have to be an administrator to be a successful leader.

Motivation is seen as an internal system from which the leadership style of an individual emanates. Leadership style is closely related to the communication process, which, in turn, influences the extent to which one is able to affect the behavior of others in order to achieve group goals.

Since goal orientation is so important to leadership, it would seem that some basic understanding of the types of organizational goals would be of value to those in leadership positions.

It is no less important for leaders in nursing education to have a working knowledge of the relationships between goal attainment and organizational norms, organizational norms and power, and power and leadership. Furthermore, these relationships should be perceived as resulting in normal organizational behavior—perhaps not always totally responsible organizational behavior—but normal (to be expected). The conflict and competition so often described in organizations is generally built into the system and cannot be avoided. What is abnormal, in some instances, is the manner in which leaders can or cannot cope with the conflict.

Diversity has always been a hallmark of American higher education. While one must concede that some disciplines within the system might be criticized justifiably for tending more toward sameness than toward diversity, nursing is not one of them. On the contrary, nursing programs seem to proliferate at every level of post-secondary education, from the vocational–technical level through the baccalaureate, masters, and doctoral levels. Sometimes it is difficult to distinguish goals of the various levels and, sometimes, even when goals are distinguishable, programs leading to their attainment are not. Too often counterparts in nursing service state that they cannot distinguish the end products of several educational programs and proceed to demonstrate this by making no distinction in the kinds of responsibilities they assign to nurses who are graduates of diploma, associate degree, and baccalaureate programs.

Leaders need to see nursing education as an integral part of the total system of higher education. They need to understand the impact of higher education in the role of educating individuals for every other institution in society. Broadly speaking, official goals of higher education stem from the goals set by society, as a whole. These goals then apply, in a general way, to all institutions of higher education. The point to be recognized is that the goals of nursing education are derived from the goals of higher education and, thus, are related primarily to the transmission of knowledge and only secondarily to improved health care.

In contrast to the official goals of nursing education, which are often identified in institutional documents, in position papers published by official nursing organizations, or in pronouncements by high-ranking officials in schools of nursing, operative goals are more often identified by observing what really goes on in a school of nursing—by looking at its by-laws, organizational chart, policies, and other such materials. As a general rule, there is an identifiable difference between official and operative goals in an organization, although both generally tend in the same direction. This difference, while frustrating to the idealist, is explained by the realist as the difference between maximizing and "satisficing" in an organization. It is assumed that in every organization official goals can only be achieved if every member exerts maximal effort. However, not every individual in an organization exerts maximal effort. Some individuals "satisfice," that is, they exert the amount of effort deemed acceptable to that organization. Thus, the degree to which an organization is involved in satisficing instead of maximizing is the degree to which there will be a difference between operative and official goals.[1] The problem presented here, which must be dealt with by persons in leadership positions, is related to the cause of satisficing. Why do people perform at a level lower than that prescribed by official goals? In general, there are three reasons given for this type of organizational behavior: (a) the individuals involved do not know what is expected of them; (b) the individuals involved do not have the necessary knowledge and/or skill to do what is expected of them;

and (c) the individuals involved do not want to do what is expected of them. Needless to say, it is easier to deal with the first two reasons than it is to deal with the third reason. However, some understanding of the causes of this behavior might help to eliminate it to some extent or to deal with it when it occurs.

When organizational goals in nursing education are examined further, it becomes evident that some of the constraints and some of the facilitators that are both external and internal to schools of nursing must be evaluated more realistically. Just a few of these variables, which may be constraining or facilitating, are money, government controls and regulations, accrediting agencies, physical facilities, contractual agreements with other agencies, admissions policies, progression policies, faculty load, curriculum development, and organizational structure.[1] Any one of the above might be a facilitating or a constraining factor in achieving organizational goals and thus affect the degree of success or failure the leader experiences. In light of these factors, it is essential that realistic goals be set. To do otherwise is to build in frustration and failure at the outset of the nursing leadership process.

Organizational norms are standards of behavior set by an organization and to which individuals adhere. The behaviors may be explicit or implicit. Explicit norms are conscious and formal. They are conscious to the extent that they may be known, that is, to the extent that they are public, and formal to the extent that they are implemented through the formal structure of the organization. Examples of explicit norms in nursing education are organizational charts and by-laws and policies governing appointment, promotion, and tenure. Implicit norms, in contrast, are unconscious and informal, that is, they are not published and are usually implemented through the informal organization. Norms such as "Don't hassle," "You scratch my back and I'll scratch yours," "You stay off my turf and I'll stay off yours," are unfortunately as common in academia as they are in profit-oriented organizations. Many implicit norms in colleges and universities have to do with the acquisition and exercise of power. Administrative leadership, therefore, is effective to the extent that an organization conforms to explicit, rather than implicit, norms.

It is important to understand the subtle differences and the relationships that exist among concepts of power, authority, and leadership. Because of the faculty role in governance, most nursing schools are administered by the exercise of power and leadership, rather than by raw authority. The sources of power are threefold: (a) position, (b) expertise, and (c) charisma. The power that comes from position is akin to formal authority. It emanates from the position, not from the individual. Expertise, as a source of power, is relative to one's position within the formal structure of the organization and is also relative to the needs of that organization at a given time. An important point to remember with regard to expertise in administration is that the expert skill to be desired is administrative as opposed to technical. This is based on the premise that as one moves up within the organizational structure, proportionately more time is spent in administrative (planning, organizing, directing, and controlling) than in technical activities (directly related to organizational output). Assuming this to be true, then as one moves up within the formal structure, it becomes necessary to acquire the administrative skills that are a requirement of the position and to relinquish some of the technical skills that previously served as a source of expertise and, therefore, of power. Charisma refers to those personal characteristics that serve to induce others to follow. To the extent that position, expertise, and charisma reside in the same individual, that individual is powerful in an organization.

While recognizing that an assessment of traits and characteristics is not the most sophisticated approach to the study of leadership, Kazmier identifies the following as repeatedly appearing in the literature related to leadership: (a) intelligence, (b) the ability to assess group goals, and (c) good interpersonal relationships. For leadership to evolve, these must appear in concert (the absence of one cannot be offset by the presence, to a greater degree, of another), and they must be possessed to a greater extent than by other individuals in the group.[2] The leader in nursing education is a potentially powerful person in society. Whether this potential is realized depends, in part, on the individual's effectiveness in implementing the leadership process both within and outside the school of nursing.

As institutions of higher education become more complex, greater leadership ability is required to make them function more effectively. In this quest for effective leadership, the findings of research tend to point more and more to the importance of sensitivity and insight into the needs of the total situation in which the leader is to function. The identification of essential leadership qualities per se will not ensure effective results unless these qualities are determined in relation to a specific organizational situation and unless their functioning becomes an integral part of organizational behavior. This concept of leadership as a function of the situation rather than as a number of not too well-defined qualities possessed by a given individual is extremely important. Because leadership functions in a specific situation relative to a specific group of people, those who aspire to success in positions of leadership need to develop an understanding of group culture and its complexities.

In view of the leadership role in which nursing educators find themselves, it is important that they skillfully use some basic concepts of group behavior relative to the leadership process. The three dimensions of organizational behavior—the group task, the individual and his personal needs, and the interpersonal relationships among group members as they work toward a common goal—create a complex situation. Because of the faculty role in governance in institutions of higher education, most schools of nursing have a complex committee structure that feeds into the decision-making process at various levels of the organization. As a result, most faculty members, whether or not they are in administrative positions, find themselves called upon to assume the leadership role at some time. In addition to assuming leadership roles within the school of nursing, educators are called upon to exercise leadership with other groups within the institution of higher education and with other professional and/or community groups. In these situations, the educators may be called upon to function as expert practitioners, researchers, or consultants.

In order for the leadership process to be implemented successfully, a new premium must be placed on better planned and more effective communication. In fact, communication is probably the human process most crucial to effective leadership. Fortunately, one of the easiest processes to observe is how people communicate with each other, particularly in face-to-face situations. This does not imply that the process is simple—quite the contrary. The information transferred during the process is often highly variable and complex. Facts, feelings, innuendos, and perceptions are communicated in a single message. Not only do persons communicate verbally, but they communicate through postures and gestures, tones of voice, and other behaviors related to communication style.[3]

The simplest analysis of communication is to answer the questions: "Who communicates with whom?" "How often?" "For how long?" For what purpose?" Implied in the foregoing discussion is the idea that nursing educators communicate with several categories of individuals and groups both outside and within the educational community and organization. To answer the proposed questions in a specific way, it would be necessary to look at the communication patterns of nursing educators and to analyze them in terms of:

I. Outside the university community (any person or persons other than students not included in the formal organizational structure of the educational institution)
   A. Individual
      (1) purpose
      (2) time
   B. Group
      (1) purpose
      (2) time
II. Inside the university organization (any person or persons included in the formal organizational structure of the educational institution)
   A. Upward communication (to an organizational level higher than that of the communicator)
      (1) Individual
         (a) purpose
         (b) time
      (2) Group
         (a) purpose
         (b) time
   B. Downward communication (to an organizational level lower than that of the communicator)
      (1) Individual
         (a) purpose
         (b) time

(2) Group
   (a) purpose
   (b) time
C. Lateral communication (to the same organizational level as that of the communicator)
   (1) Individual
      (a) purpose
      (b) time
   (2) Group
      (a) purpose
      (b) time
III. Students
   A. Undergraduate
      (1) Individual
         (a) purpose
         (b) time
      (2) Group
         (a) purpose
         (b) time
   B. Graduate
      (1) Individual
         (a) purpose
         (b) time
      (2) Group
         (a) purpose
         (b) time

In the above outline, individual communication is defined as communication with one person at a time; group communication is defined as communication with more than one person at a time.

This kind of analysis would enable one to describe the quantitative aspects of formal communication patterns of nursing educators, and would give some indication of the nature, scope, and time consumed by face-to-face verbal communication in nursing education. It would be more difficult to observe all of the spontaneous, informal communications of the educator/leader, but it is assumed that informal communication, at all levels, is frequent.

In the nursing leadership process (noted in Fig. 1, page 96), communication is portrayed as essential to all components of the process. In order to get at the notion of effective communication, one must make other observations about the communication process of nursing educators as they communicate in group and individual situations. Although it is important to spend sufficient time in communication with many groups and individuals, both outside and inside the educational setting, it is also important that the quality of communication be sufficient to bring about the desired goal through deciding, relating, influencing, and facilitating in a given situation. In this respect, it is often helpful to observe patterns of "triggering" in groups. This refers to who talks after whom (who triggers whom and in what ways), and whether this communication reflects support (encouragement) or nonsupport (undoing). Observations of this kind of overt surface behavior provide clues as to what is happening between and among people beneath the surface.[3] It is a partial indicator of who decides for whom, who relates with whom, who influences whom, and who facilitates what.

Another kind of communication behavior that can be observed is "who interrupts whom?" Observing this kind of behavior can give some indication of how individuals perceive their own status of power within a group relative to the status or power of other group members.[3] It would be interesting to make these kinds of observations in a multidisciplinary group of professional educators. Perhaps it would give some indication of the extent to which nursing educators have actualized their power potential.

Communication style (whether a person is assertive, questioning, humorous; whether his voice is loud, soft, grating; whether he uses gestures) is important to the leadership process in terms of the possible effects of a given communication style on the individuals with whom the person is communicating. There is much in the literature today about assertiveness and how assertive behavior can lead to influence and power within a group. Although there are many situations in which one must be assertive in order to exercise leadership, there are other situations in which this style of communicating causes others to "tune out" the leader, thus causing the leader's influence in the group to decline.[3]

In addition to the above, more readily observable, characteristics of the communication process, there are other, less easily observed characteristics. These are levels of communication and filtering. It is important for the leader to be aware of the subtleties and complications in levels of communication so that communication channels not ordinarily used can be opened. It is common in nursing education for faculty members to express feelings of anger, frustration, or futility, to each other privately, but never to share those feelings with the people who elicit them. This situation is frequently encountered during the process of curriculum development, when faculty members are experiencing feelings of insecurity, confusion, and just plain overload. In this situation the leader must be sensitive to the feelings of the group and to help them to deal with these feelings in a realistic way. When these feelings are not dealt with in an open manner, the faculty member tends to displace anger or tends to withdraw (physically or psychologically) from the situation. This kind of negative behavior is akin to throwing the proverbial "match in the haystack." It spreads like wildfire! Although this example is used to show that the leader should create an environment in which open communication can take place and that emotional issues need to be dealt with, it is also related to the more substantive issue of setting realistic goals and reassessing them periodically.

Filtering is a process whereby both the sender and receiver decide what they will send and what they will receive based on a number of factors, including self-image, image of others in the situation, definition of the situation, motives, feelings, intentions and attitudes, and expectations of themselves and others in the situation.[3] These factors make it possible for communication to break down, since much data related to these factors is personal and is not revealed to others.

Communication patterns vary widely in different types of organizational settings. Most institutions of higher education are organized according to the pluralistic, collegial model. This type of structure is a modification of the monocratic, bureaucratic concept, providing for a pluralistic sharing of powers to make policy and program decisions on a collegial basis. Under this type of structure, there are many channels of communication. Two-way communication operates through a vertical channel, but communication is also circular and horizontal. Given this freedom of communication, the opportunity for beneficial interactions is greater than it is in an organization where great emphasis is placed on vertical channels.[4]

McGregor believed that the kinds of underlying assumptions a leader makes about people will determine how he leads them. For example, McGregor's Theory X is seen as a traditional model of superior–subordinate direction and control. In this model, it is assumed that man works for money, that he is basically lazy and will avoid work whenever he can, and, thus, that he must be closely supervised and controlled by economic incentives. In contrast to Theory X, Theory Y assumes that work is as natural to man as rest and play, that man has a hierarchy of needs and as lower order needs are satisfied, higher order needs predominate. In this model, control is seen as self-control, and the role of the leader is to provide an environment or climate in which subordinates are permitted to use their talents.[5] An analogy might be made between the extremes of the range of leadership behavior developed by Tannenbaum and Schmidt and by McGregor's Theory X and Theory Y. The range of leadership behavior describes the action alternatives available to a leader in structuring an interpersonal situation for decision making. The range is from total leader authority on one end to total group autonomy on the other. In boss-centered leadership, the leader simply makes the decision and announces it. In subordinate-centered leadership, the leader permits subordinates to function within limits he has defined. Boss-centered leadership characterizes the leader who maintains a high degree of control, whereas subordinate-centered leadership characterizes a leader who relinquishes a high degree of control. Each type of action described between the extremes is related to the degree of authority used by the leader and the amount of freedom available to his subordinates in reaching decisions.[6] Boss-centered leadership is characteristic of Theory X leaders and subordinate-centered leadership characterizes the Theory Y leader. Herzberg's research on job satisfaction substantiates the theory that the motivation to work is based on the satisfaction of man's highest order of needs. Factors identified by Herzberg as motivators are achievement, recognition, work itself, responsibility, and advancement. This would seem to be true, particularly, for professionals in educational settings.[7]

In addition to an awareness of motivational factors that lead to goal attainment, the leader needs to be familiar with the relationship among morale, motivation, and productivity, if one is to create an environment that will enhance goal attainment. Morale refers to the extent to which an individual is able to satisfy personal needs within the context of the organization. Productivity refers to the satisfaction of organizational goals. Negative motivational techniques are those that reduce the opportunity an individual has to satisfy personal needs. Positive motivational techniques are those that increase the opportunity an individual has to satisfy his personal needs. Therefore, negative motivational techniques always result in low morale, whereas positive motivational techniques always result in high morale. Only to the extent that the satisfaction of personal needs is congruent with the satisfaction of organizational goals is there a positive relationship between high morale and high productivity. When factors in the work situation itself serve to meet the personal needs of the individual, high morale leads to high productivity. If the individual is permitted a high degree of personal need satisfaction extraneous to the requirements of the job, then high morale and low productivity coexist. Low morale, on the other hand, may combine with high productivity for a short period of time, provided there is something that binds the individual to the organization. However, over the long term, low morale leads to low productivity.

Morale, motivation, and productivity provide clues to the environment the leader in nursing education needs to structure in order to achieve predetermined goals. There is considerable evidence that faculty members are more productive in pluralistic collegial organizations than in monocratic, bureaucratic organizations. Therefore, one might expect leaders in nursing education to create an environment in which (a) leadership is not confined to those holding status positions in the power echelon, (b) good human relations are considered essential to group production and to meeting the needs of individual members of the group, (c) responsibility, as well as power and authority, can be shared, (d) those affected by a program or policy share in decision making with respect to that program or policy, (e) the individual finds security in a dynamic climate in which he shares responsibility for decision making, (f) unity of purpose is secured through consensus and group loyalty, (g) maximum production is attained in a threat-free climate, (h) the line and staff organization is used to divide labor and implement policies and programs developed by the total group affected, (i) the situation and not the position determines the right and privilege to exercise leadership, (j) the individual in the organization is not expendable, and (k) evaluation is a group responsibility.[8] Presumably, this kind of environment would promote high morale and high productivity and, therefore, allow the educational leader to experience considerable success.

Successful leadership in nursing education is complex and depends to a large extent on knowledge of and skill in implementing the leadership process. Its effect is based in the motivational system of both leader and follower(s). Nursing educators have a unique opportunity to exercise leadership in a variety of situations, both inside and outside the university. Not only do they have the opportunity to influence students in their own schools of nursing, but by participating in research, continuing education and consultation, their influence may be even more widespread. Faculty in graduate programs in nursing have an even greater opportunity to influence large numbers of individuals through the efforts of graduates of the programs who, in turn, assume influential positions in nursing. Administrators in schools of nursing bear a special responsibility for exercising leadership in relation to their faculties, since people tend to lead in the manner in which they are led.

Nursing educators need to develop a power base (a) within the system of higher education, (b) within the nursing profession itself, and (c) within the community, and thence the larger society. In order to do this, nursing education needs to:

1. Educate more nurses at the doctoral level;
2. Encourage its members to engage in scholarly research and publish the findings;
3. Establish a collegial relationship with nursing service and other health disciplines;
4. Place more stress on the development of leadership and political skills; curriculum should include both a theory base and practice in

the processes related to leadership and power, including intergroup conflict resolution and team building;
5. Expand continuing education programs.

THE NURSING LEADERSHIP PROCESS IN NURSING SERVICE AND INSERVICE EDUCATION

Elizabeth Ozimek Kaye

Nursing leadership has been defined as the process of deciding, relating, influencing, and facilitating the behavior of other persons in their effort toward goal setting and achievement. Permeating this process is communication, which results in change.

This process is part of every function of every professional nurse. Each nurse, during the course of the work day, will decide, relate, influence, and facilitate the behavior of peers, patients, auxiliary and interdisciplinary personnel through communication to achieve the goals of the institution and nursing service. The educational preparation of the professional nurse will influence the breadth, depth, and consistency of the process of nursing leadership.

The leadership process in nursing service is complex. The new staff nurse finds herself involved in the leadership process on her very first day of work. She will be deciding, relating, influencing, and facilitating the behavior of licensed practical nurses and attendants in most instances. She does not become a great leader overnight. Leadership research has disproved the leader-trait approach stipulating that leaders are born and has revealed the importance of the situational-interaction approach to leadership.[1] Very often the situations the nurse may find herself a part of, in the hospital-institutional setting, tend to suppress the expression of her leadership behavior. Many nurses continually point out that frequently they are not consulted or involved in decision making and policy establishment regarding nursing care. The complaint often heard from nursing staff is that they do not understand why a certain personnel policy was established, yet they must transmit and translate it to their staff and attendants.

Too often the nursing staff complains that they must provide care to patients under conditions that hinder the quality of nursing care because they were not consulted during the decision-making, planning, and organizational process of a proposed change.

Hagen and Wolff's research study of nursing leadership behavior revealed findings of great significance to those involved in nursing service in the hospital setting. They studied the leadership behaviors, both effective and ineffective, of the director of nursing service, supervisor of nurses, and head nurse. Communication seemed to be cited in many portions of the study and how it affects all concerned. They mentioned that the "director of nursing service in a general hospital holds the top position in nursing, yet one looks in vain for any evidence that the director of nursing service either attempts to develop a unified philosophy of nursing within her hospital or attempts to interpret nursing as a profession to people outside the nursing service department." [2] They go on to relate that there appeared to be a general lack of a "sense of unity and we-ness, either within the nursing service department as a whole or within the hospital as a whole. There is little evidence that the director of nursing service provides leadership to promote a feeling of belonging to a large institution or to the profession of nursing as a whole." [2] Leadership behavior must be examined by all and the elusive "they," frequently mentioned, must be isolated, examined, and analyzed before nursing can improve patient care and provide appropriate leadership. Hagen and Wolff state that the "absence of long-range planning and the development of an *espirit de corps* among nurses is probably related to the fact that the incidents collected indicated that subordinates tended to reflect very little understanding of the next highest superior's role in the hospital." [3] Coupled with this finding was that "incidents also gave the impression that most directors of nursing service see no real point in explaining their decisions or actions to subordinates, nor do most of them either seek or accept suggestions from subordinates. Perhaps the director of nursing service has not had any training in communication or has had inadequate training so that she feels insecure in determining when, what, and how much to explain to subordinates." [3] Supervisors, as well, recognized, in this research study, that very often "they should have explained their actions to subordinates, but excused their failure to do so on the basis that they were too busy or short of staff." [4] Supervisors as well as directors "react to the symptom rather than to the basic problem." [5] The lack of problem-solving ability was noted as a negative point in leadership behavior. Deciding is the beginning point in the leadership process. Hagen and Wolf feel that the inability to perform leadership behavior might have been due to the poor educational backgrounds of the supervisors.

The head nurse, in the hospital, very often is the relator, influencer, and facilitator of decision making. Of course she makes decisions, also, but she is the prime communicator of policies and procedures from nursing and hospital administration. She sets the climate for acceptance and motivation. She is the vital change agent. It appears that in most agencies she works with the largest number of personnel—nursing service personnel and multidisciplinary personnel. In most agencies, it is the head nurse and the staff nurse, who display the leadership behaviors of deciding, relating, influencing, and facilitating the behavior of others. These nurses have the greatest impact on the behavior of patients. The clinical supervisor or specialist nursing practitioner offers guidance and consultation regarding patient care thereby implementing the components of leadership behavior in their relationships with the head nurse and staff nurses.

Nursing practitioners decide, relate, influence, and facilitate quality patient care, nursing service, and institutional goal achievement. However, the leadership behavior of "deciding" in the realm of policy making that affects day-to-day functioning appears to be a limited area for nursing personnel. Hagen and Wolff found limitations in the "deciding" behavior in terms of the "reluctance or inability to analyze a problem situation" by directors of nursing service and supervisors.[6] Since there is overlapping of functions, all nursing practitioners displayed limitations in "doing long-range planning and problem solving." [7]

Further and continued research needs to be undertaken in the area of nursing service. Through this research, nursing service personnel can look at their practice, at their strengths and weaknesses, and at the precipitating and perpetuating factors causing problems related to the delivery of quality nursing service.

How can the nursing leadership process be augmented and strengthened to improve the quality of patient care provided by nursing service personnel? Part of the answer to this question, but certainly not a panacea, is the development of staff through a well-planned and well-executed inservice education program. Nursing's major concern continues to be a lack of sufficient numbers of educationally qualified generalist and specialist nursing practitioners in the hospital setting. Proper formal preparation must precede continuing and inservice education. Cooper states that inservice education is one facet of continuing nursing education and its importance cannot be overestimated. "It is the educational opportunities provided by the employer for the employee to attain or improve his capabilities." [8] The nursing leadership process components of deciding, relating, influencing, and facilitating surround and incorporate the entire inservice education program, beginning with a base of institutional and nursing service goal determination and culminating with institutional and nursing service goal achievement. These leadership behaviors are a dynamic process, occurring between the inservice educator and learner through communication that results in charge.

Institutional and nursing service goal determination form the base of the inservice education program. It must determine where nursing practice is going and why it is where it is. Are the goals of the nursing service department compatible and related to those of the patients and those of the institution? These goals must be based on standards for person-centered and family-centered nursing care. The task of each employee will ultimately be the achievement of these goals. The goals will define *parameters* and give direction to nursing service personnel and to the inservice education program. Functions or job descriptions emerge from these goals and serve as the basis for action. Functions may overlap, but there are unique functions for each member of a health care agency. Besides job descriptions, agency policies and procedures also give direction. When the task of deciding goals has been accomplished, the process of inservice education begins.

The goal of inservice education is to improve the work performance of the adult worker. Concepts of andragogy, as reviewed by Tobin, Yoder, Hull, and Scott, stipulate that the inservice educator must be aware of the adult learner's needs and know how to respond to them.[9] The teaching of adults is unique and cannot be implemented in the same way that children are taught. Knowledge of adult learning will assist the inservice educator in deciding, relating, influencing, and facilitating the development of the nursing service employee. Some statements about adult characteristics cited by Tobin, et al reveal that "Adults must want to learn and must feel the need for a particular knowledge or skill." [9] Motivation is the key. The employee requires ego satisfaction and it is the aware educator who knows the learners, makes use of their desires, remembers Maslow's hierarchy of needs, and includes their participation when involved in deciding and planning the program.

Another statement is, "Adults prefer learning based on active involvement and the actual problems they face in their working environment." [9] They do not learn well through a rigid lecture method or when faced with environmental annoyances. The "real" world is where they are and where they must function. They want guidance in coping with it. Teaching methods using such approaches as the critical-incident technique, problem-solving group tasks, role-playing, and clinical teaching by the clinical nurse expert all permit active participation of the adult learner. The adult learner also must be given the opportunity to question and the freedom to disagree in an environment that allows for mature relationships. It is important for the inservice educator to communicate to nursing personnel that their opinions and criticisms are noteworthy in what unfortunately might be a bureaucratic structure in which the nurse's opinions are rarely sought in policy making. Fear may also be a result of internalized childhood learning experiences where the teacher did the talking and the student remained passive and listened. How learning is communicated and the degree to which it will influence the individual's "self" will determine whether change will occur. Another characteristic of the adult is that he wants guidance and wants to know how he is progressing. An employee will want to know what is expected of him—what his role is in the organization and how he fits in; what are the policies and procedures and how do they affect him. Employees expect to have their performances evaluated and expect that the inservice educator will be aware of individual differences in their preservice education, perceptions, and experiences. Adults prefer an informal setting when learning. The individuals involved in the experience with them are their peers and co-workers. The inservice educator is a peer, a co-worker, and a leader. All learn from the shared experiences and these should transmit a feeling of worth or security. To threaten worth and security would narrow perception and diminish learning considerably.

Knowledge of the goals of the institution and of nursing service, and knowledge of the learners and their needs help the inservice educator to decide upon objectives for and the design of the program. The program is also determined by the organizational and administrative structure of the nursing inservice education department. In order to achieve a program that continually develops and refines the nurse's leadership behavior from the moment of her employment, there must be a sound base from which the process can emerge.

Models for Department of Nursing Inservice Education

There are various models of a nursing inservice education department. The department may be (a) centralized, (b) decentralized, or (c) a combination of a centralized-decentralized structure. A centralized structure is one in which the coordinator of nursing inservice education is a position in line with that of the director of nursing services, or is one with status equal to that of the assistant director of nursing service. The American Nurses Association has designated that the nursing inservice education coordinator should possess a master's degree in nursing.[10] Ideally the functional areas of preparation should be inservice education administration and a specialty in a specific clinical nursing area. The relationship of the coordinator of nursing inservice education in the organizational structure is one that is still being clarified in most agencies. Unfortunately it appears that in most instances an unprepared assistant director of nursing services is delegated this assignment, due to interest or to the administrator's view that someone must do this, rather than a nurse with advanced education and experience in the field of nursing inservice education. The line position giving equal status to director of nursing services and a coordinator of nursing inservice education is desirable.

Today the centralized model of inservice education may also take on a broader range, which is considered best and which is the general organizational plan in most large medical centers. This model is slowly emerging in smaller hospitals because of realization that professional continuing education is important. This broader approach to the centralized model views the *nursing* inservice education department as only *one* of the various disciplines' inservice departments. In this approach nursing inservice education is part of the entire hospital's inservice education system wherein each discipline provides its own program with its own specified inservice education administrator and instructors. The coordinator of this centralized model should be an educator with a doctoral degree in education, who is well versed in adult education, and can coordinate all inservice activities through a multidisciplinary committee. This committee should comprise each discipline's inservice education department administrator who, with commensurate authority, is responsible for its particular program. This approach fosters ease of communication among the various departments, thus facilitating institutional goal achievement. The coordinator acts as chairman of the multidisciplinary committee, the primary responsibility of which is multidisciplinary general orientation and continuing inservice education programming. Each discipline's inservice department administrator formulates, on an annual basis, the purpose, philosophy, objectives, and complete inservice program for the department. The nursing inservice education department program should include participation in the multidisciplinary general orientation, a specific role orientation course, skill development—intellectual, behavioral and manual—unit administration and clinical specialty inservice development, and continuing *nursing* inservice education, as well as participation in *multidisciplinary* continuing inservice education.

The decentralized model of the nursing inservice education department is generally utilized when the agency's organizational structure is also decentralized in nature—sectionalized or unitized. Here a nursing inservice educator is part of the multidisciplinary team of professionals working in a particular unit and is generally responsible to the section or unit chief who may or may not be a nurse.

The nurse instructor's primary responsibility in this instance is the complete range of nursing inservice programming as mentioned above, based on the needs of the unit nursing staff and unit goals. There also may be a multidisciplinary committee or team of professionals offering continuing inservice education to all agency staff on a regular basis. This model is viewed as having some limitations in terms of the communication process among various units or sections when each plans and implements its own nursing inservice education program. Duplication of effort and cost factors may present negative values in some instances.

The third model for a nursing inservice education department is a combination centralized-decentralized model and is viewed as being the most desirable in maintaining and improving the work performance of nursing service employees. This approach offers formal centralized programs, beginning with multidisciplinary general orientation, role orientation, selected intellectual behavior and manual skill development, selected unit inservice administration, and continuing inservice education programs (see Fig. 4—Situational Aspects of Nursing Leadership Process in Inservice Education).

Common learner needs relevant to the nursing service staff involved must be determined. *Formal* courses, or classes, incorporating nursing theory and clinical practice are continuously offered by inservice instructors who are located at the institution's designated nursing inservice education department. *Informal* courses and classes would also be offered to nursing service personnel, but take place solely at the employee's assigned clinical area—the decentralized component of this model. The specific, clinically assigned, inservice instructor, head nurse, supervisor, and specialist nursing practitioner, who demonstrate expertise in the particular clinical nursing specialty, act as role models. The nursing inservice education coordinator offers guidance and acts as consultant and resource person to nurse instructors in the decentralized model. Both formal and informal programming is coordinated by the nursing inservice education coordinator. This third model, with the inclusion of the multidisciplinary inservice education coordinator and multidisciplinary continuing education committee, seems to be the most favorable today.

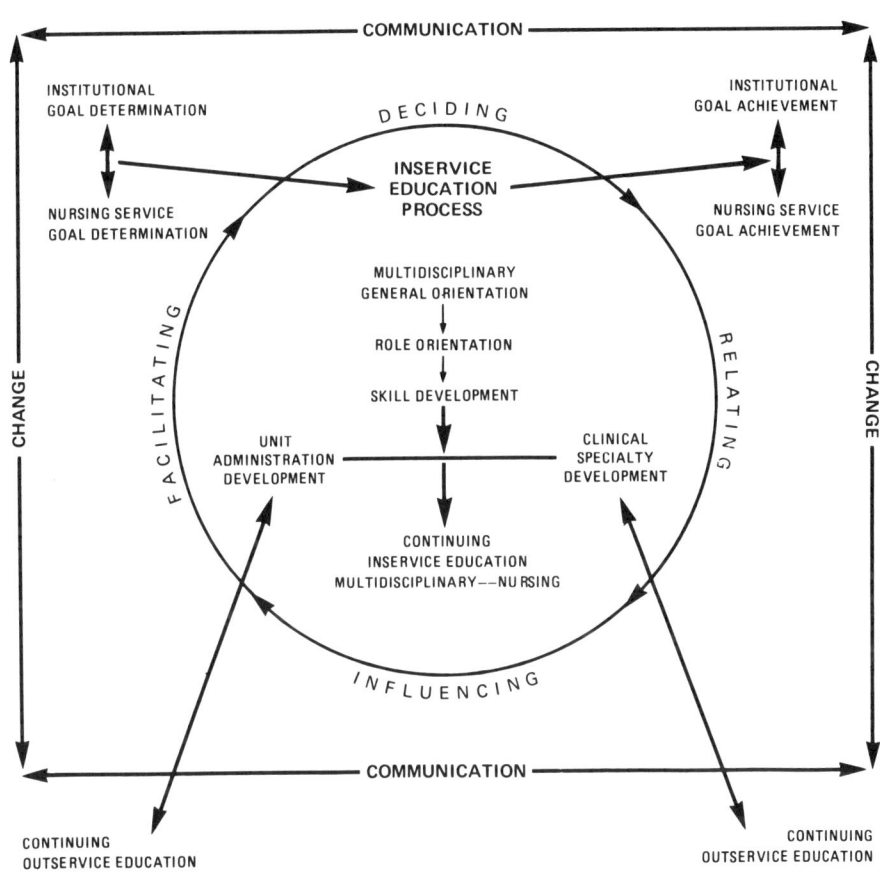

FIG. 4 Situational Aspects of the Nursing Leadership Process in Inservice Education.

All three models of nursing inservice education departments require a thorough analysis of learning needs employing such techniques as questionnaires, skill inventories, interviews, observation, job histories, and records and reports for appropriate programming. Other resources to analyze needs are various established nursing service committees, such as procedures, policies, audit, research, medication, staff development, records and forms analysis, and any other committees particular to an agency's needs. The members of these committees should be representative of all practitioner levels. These invaluable assessment mechanisms will permit programming that is motivating, timely, and that meets the needs of patients, nurse learners, and the institution.

Use of established parameters, as previously mentioned—the philosophy, goals and objectives of the institution, of nursing service and nursing inservice education; job descriptions and their relationships; policies and procedures manuals; the tables and charts of organization; preservice education and job histories of the learners; practice standards of care—particularly the American Nurses Association standards of nursing practice, ie, the five American Nurses Association Divisions of Practice Standards, and the Joint Commission on Accreditation of Hospital Standards for Nursing Services; and finally, the results of retrospective outcome studies of care, all serve to aid the inservice educator in determining learning and practice deficits and in planning needed courses and classes.

Nursing leadership behaviors are developed and enhanced through the active involvement of nursing staff in the planning of programs. The nursing staff, along with the inservice educator, will be deciding, relating, influencing, and facilitating during this first phase of each course and class; that is, operationalizing these components and using them as guidelines in program planning and implementation.

Curriculum Aspects of the Inservice Education

Although the curriculum aspects of inservice education appear to be sequential, this may not be the case if the learner's needs and institutional needs do not warrant such development. The multidisciplinary general orientation course is usually the beginning point of the inservice education process. Depending upon the organizational model, this course may be coordinated by the institution's inservice education director, multidisciplinary staff development coordinator, personnel director, nursing inservice education coordinator, or the multidisciplinary department heads with an elected committee chairman. At this time the purpose, behavioral objectives, and complete design of the course is accomplished. This first impression and feeling tone of the institution is a lasting one. Since it is multidisciplinary in nature, it must meet the needs of all new employees in all departments and services. The purpose of the general orientation is to familiarize the new employee with the philosophy and objectives of the agency, the physical plant, and the table or chart of organization citing specific names of department heads, personnel policies, and the goals and objectives of each department. If possible, this general orientation should be presented to the employee on the first day or days of employment. Generally, this is not the case due to the employment process of the agency. Most frequently new personnel may begin their employment on any day of the week and it would not be economically (time and cost) feasible to present such a program frequently. If this is a problem, it must be thoroughly discussed with the personnel department, since it is most advantageous from an educational standpoint to employ personnel on a regular schedule, such as once per month, so that the general orientation program can be consistently and appropriately scheduled.

The multidisciplinary staff development committee or coordinator will execute the mechanics of the program. The coordinator will schedule department heads or their representatives to speak to the group of new employees. Some agencies use audiovisual materials, such as videotaping, 16-mm film, or sound slides that feature department heads and the physical plant thereby providing information through a time-saving method. It does not, however, replace the human factor of personally meeting individuals and the feeling of acceptance a new employee desires and receives. It is also advantageous to assist the employee in becoming familiar with the physical environment of the agency by an actual walking tour. This offers the employee the opportunity to meet as many persons as possible. A map is also a helpful handout at this time. Another very valuable handout is an "Employee's Manual," which may include all of the information received in class, in written form, for future reference. Since there is so much that a new employee must assimilate, and much is generally forgotten, a manual would reinforce information and would prevent needed information from being lost. The table or chart of organization, cited in the manual, should also provide blank spaces in which names of personnel can be written as a reminder and reference. The evaluation process begins when the multidisciplinary general orientation has been completed. A questionnaire can be devised for evaluative purposes, with both open-ended questions and a rating scale; it should be distributed to the new employee as soon as the course is completed and then administered again after three to six months of employment. Distribution of the evaluation form at time intervals permits the employee to evaluate the course and offer immediate reactions, and evaluate it through the eyes and feelings of one more experienced. The primary purpose of the general orientation course evaluation is to find out from the employee if the program presented is adequate and, if not, how the program can be improved.[11] Department heads should reevaluate the program at least annually. The evaluation forms are used as an assessment tool and, if possible, interview data, incident reports, or records, which would determine if course objectives have been met and would reflect upon the appropriateness of material presented should also be included. Program revision would then be initiated by the coordinator and designed by the multidisciplinary group as deemed necessary.

Personnel, according to their specific disciplines, should then receive a role orientation course. In nursing inservice, separate role orientation programs should be designed for professional and nonprofessional nursing service personnel. The professional role orientation program and its relationship to the nursing leadership process in nursing service follows.

Role orientation should include both formal and informal teaching. A list of the names of newly employed professional nurses is received from nursing service administration. If nurses are hired on a weekly rather than a monthly basis, a course should be offered at regular intervals. The length of the course depends upon the needs of the learner and the institution. Some agencies offer a minimum two-week and others a one-year course. All generally state their purpose is to assist newly employed nurses, with varied backgrounds in education and experience, to become familiar with the philosophy and objectives of their unit, its physical environment, and their function through a planned course provided by nursing inservice education and nursing service personnel. Demographic data on which to base an individualized role orientation course must be determined. Preservice nursing educational and experiential backgrounds are so varied that information must be gathered in order to meet the learning needs of the individual nurse. Generally, agencies can and do devise a questionnaire and checklist to obtain this information. It is advisable that the questionnaire be completed the first day and a carbon copy sent to the area supervisor for use and information. Questions should include such basic data as name, address, work assignment, licensure date, preservice education, clinical nursing experience, and administrative experience with regard to type and numbers of personnel directed. The level of mastery in the use of the nursing process appropriate to educational preparation of the nursing practitioner must be determined. A checklist inventory of acquired knowledge and nursing care procedures previously performed by the nurse should be completed at this time to prepare for the next phase of the inservice process. This inventory could be formulated in column form to check on the required content and whether a refresher or demonstration course will be necessary. Open-ended questions should report information related to what the nurse feels are her greatest areas of knowledge and skill, strengths, weaknesses, and future desires or plans in her nursing career. This provides the inservice educator and supervisor with added insight and data that aid in meeting the nurse's learning needs and serve as a base for future individualized inservice programming.

The job description, appropriate to the practitioner level of the nurse at the agency, and a nursing service orientation manual are used as standards for the role orientation course. Critical behaviors of the nurse's role should be stated so that future performance evaluation can be accomplished. Role expectations of other personnel on the unit, those above and below on the organizational table or chart, are also defined so that the nurse has a clear understanding of how all personnel work together for institutional and nursing service goal achievement. Nursing service policies and their interpretation are reviewed to show their relationship to role. This portion of the role orientation course can be formally offered by the nursing inservice educator. An introduction to or further development of the leadership behaviors of deciding, relating, influencing, and facilitating should begin at this time for professional nurses. Role orientation to the nursing process, group planning, and communication employing intellectual action-oriented techniques specifically related to the employee's role are offered. These areas would be discussed in depth in the next program phase of the nursing inservice education process. Since it is believed that the leadership process is inherent in the nurse's role, these behaviors are viewed as part of her function and should be included during this course.

The unit orientation or informal segment of the role orientation course should be designed and offered by unit personnel, preferably the supervisor or head nurse. It is thought advantageous to interweave formal class and informal orientation during each day of the role orientation course. Unit orientation should be offered on the shift during which the nurse will be practicing. If rotation of shifts is the practice, the nurse should be oriented to the unit on all shifts. A teaching guide can be prepared by the staff development committee and nursing inservice coordinator for use by unit supervisors, head nurses, or other staff. Specific unit orientation should help the nurse become familiar with the overall environment of the unit, the system of communication, and varied resources—persons, materials, and equipment. If rotation among units is the practice of the agency, the nurse should be scheduled to receive orientation to each clinical unit area appropriate to her assignment in the agency.

An evaluation questionnaire should be administered after the role orientation program has been completed and three and/or six months following employment. An interview conducted by the nursing inservice coordinator is also a valuable evaluative tool. The purpose will be to elucidate the realism, scope, and appropriateness of the course as compared to actual day-to-day functioning. Did the course prepare the nurse for her functions in the agency as seen by her immediately following the program and at a later date after she had been functioning in her role for a period of time?

Role orientation courses should be offered to the new nurse employee as well as to newly promoted or unit transferred nurses. Again functional change is involved and an orientation to prepare her to assume new functions cannot be overlooked.

Closely following the role orientation course for the nurse in the nursing inservice program is the skill development phase. Many inservice departments incorporate skill development as part of the general orientation course for professional nursing practitioners and the general orientation course for nonprofessional personnel. Skill development, including intellectual, behavioral, and manual skills, require both formal and informal teaching. The orientation questionnaire, with a skill checklist, is utilized at this time. Also, a pretest, which includes items concerning the nursing theory, behavioral skills, and manual nursing procedures, can be administered to the nurse. The individualized nature of this phase is vital to meet the needs of a particular nurse and agency. The duration of this phase again depends upon the needs of the nurse, her role expectations, her units(s) assignment, and the facility. Skill training also often includes pharmacology. By using the nursing procedure and policy manuals as teaching aids, the inservice educator can introduce them to the nurse. Perhaps these manuals will then be used for reference rather than collect dust on the shelves of nursing stations, as seems to be the case in some agencies. Providing the nurse with copies of procedures and policies appropriate to the skills discussed also helps her to retain the information since she can use the manuals for reference.

Manual skill training is complex, since "each manufacturer produces a machine that is slightly different from the competitor's product." [12] Therefore, a nurse may have used similar equipment, but may still require orientation to the agency's equipment. The inservice educator can show the nurse how to use this equipment in a simulated clinical unit in the inservice education department. The purpose, equipment, procedure, and principles, as well as points of emphasis, can be thoroughly discussed in an unhurried, quiet, and secure milieu. Once this base of review of initial knowledge is accomplished, the inservice educator should demonstrate the procedures on the nurse's assigned clinical unit, using the equipment. This facilitates transfer of learning. The introduction to equipment can also be accomplished by unit personnel. The nurse would then be assigned specific patient care to give her the opportunity to perform the procedures under the guidance of inservice instructor, supervisor, or head nurse. The manual skill inventory portion of the orientation questionnaire would be checked as having been completed when each manual skill is performed satisfactorily.

Continued introduction to the nursing leadership process in role orientation can be further developed at this time. Principles of adult education, as mentioned previously, with regard to the presentation of material to enhance transfer of learning must be considered in light of the educational experience of each practitioner. The "deciding" component of leadership behavior can be discussed in terms of a review of organization theory, setting priorities, exercising judgment, and the entire area of decision making. The "relating" component would involve a discussion of communication types, barriers, and the effects upon relationships with personnel. "Influencing" others would involve a discussion of group dynamics—types and functions, and motivation. The leadership behavior component, "facilitating," should be included in discussing problem solving and the management of change. Intellectual and behavior skill development is most certainly as important as manual skill development for the new employee. However, role orientation cannot be limited to the newly employed nurse. This phase of development is so complex it must also involve reviewing and strengthening particular intellectual, behavioral, and manual skills of all nurses, since "various machines are simply not used regularly on all units" and one constantly must improve relationships among personnel.[12]

An evaluation questionnaire and post-test should be administered to the new employee when the skill development course is completed. The post-test (generally a duplication of the pretest) should reveal whether the behavioral objectives of the course have been achieved. Demonstrations of manual skill and interviews between supervisory personnel and the nurse employee will also aid in the evaluation process of this phase of the nursing inservice program.

Administration and clinical specialty development are accomplished primarily through further education in a college or university setting. When the nurse wishes to further and advance her nursing career into the area of nursing administration or nursing clinical specialization, she will require further education in an institution of higher education. When this has been accomplished and her role in the nursing service agency becomes a new one, she would participate in a role orientation course provided by the agency's nursing inservice education department, as previously discussed. Today many agencies are sponsoring continuing outservice development courses and programs in nursing colleges and universities, state nurses associations, hospitals, organizations, and health agencies, with current emphasis on continuing education in the health field. It is believed that basic nursing education prepares the nurse to function as a nursing practitioner and leader. Leadership has been defined as the process of deciding, relating, influencing, and facilitating the behavior of other persons in their effort toward goal setting and goal achievement. If the nurse wants to become a nurse administrator, clinical specialist, or inservice educator, she cannot accomplish this through the inservice education department of a health care agency, but only through further formal education.

The health care agency should provide nursing practitioners with all kinds of experience in continuing inservice or outservice education to ensure the continued development of their competence. This as well as other inservice programs serve to attain institutional and nursing service goal achievement.

With regard to continuing outservice education, it is believed that the agency must be committed to provide the nurse employee with opportunities to attend these programs. Institutional policies must be established regarding time, payment of fees, and staffing patterns, so that the nurse can attend and/or participate in such programs outside the agency. Generally, the inservice coordinator will develop a monthly continuing outservice education schedule which can be posted at various areas of the agency. This will facilitate communication and awareness of the programs. She can then relate specific information to staff and perhaps influence and motivate their attendance.

Continuing inservice education—multidisciplinary and nursing—involves extensive study of the learning needs of staff. A multidisciplinary continuing education committee provides the best base of organization. A committee structure to identify needs and plan programs will also foster motivation and program support. Continuing inservice education incorporates such programming as independent study; institutes; panel discussions; short-term courses or programs for nurses working in specialized nursing care units; nursing case study sessions; lectures; conferences on utilization of the nursing process and/or administrative themes; and workshops to continue to refine nursing leadership behavior skills, to solve specific patient problems, and to gain new knowledge. These are some examples of the types of continuing inservice programs designed to meet the learning needs of personnel. It must be stressed, however, that the objective is always to improve the abilities of individuals and their nursing performance in a particular health care agency.

Many agencies are initiating contractual agreements with local colleges and universities to provide continuing education programs, both multdisciplinary and nursing. The college university faculty is the teaching staff. Nursing students should be permitted to attend continuing inservice programs and student participation should be planned with the inservice coordinator and the faculty. Attendance of students at the inservice education program would build rapport and plant the seeds that inservice education is an important part of the work world of the nursing staff.

Administration and the patients demand that nursing staff be competent in their performance. Health care is costly and nursing service is just beginning to devise methods to audit the performance of nursing staff. Therefore, in most institutions retrospective studies of nursing care outcomes are slowly evolving. These evaluations lead to reassessment and review of the inservice education learning needs of staff. Once these learning needs are isolated, program planning, as has been briefly described, can be initiated. One factor that cannot be overlooked in any discussion of program planning is cost.

Throughout the entire inservice education process, the numbers of participants, their wages, and resources must be considered. Preparation of the annual budget for the inservice education department requires skill and is time consuming. Some institutions will have a specific outline that the nursing inservice coordinator can follow. The importance of long-range planning is reflected in planning a budget. The assistance of budget experts should be sought, if necessary, since items could be overlooked that would result in the lack of resources required to conduct programs. Some institutions are required to submit a separate budget for each proposed program. In this instance, program content and needs should be described in detail so that reviewers can understand the purposes and reasons for requests.

To provide continuity for all activities of inservice education, it is recommended that the inservice education instructors be aware and be provided with the opportunity to participate in all programs and in each activity of the inservice education department. Eng states that assigning instructors as to program and shift provides each instructor with the opportunity to participate in each activity of staff development ensuring their awareness of the total program and a high level of personal enthusiasm; provides for the continuity of activity; promotes the development of rapport with all instructors of staff development; and utilizes, most economically, the time and skills of each instructor.[13]

Another important area involved in inservice education and which aids in providing continuity for all activities of the department is records and reports. These are unique to each agency, but are important considerations since they are "designed to provide the data base for the agency's information needs. Such documents serve a specific purpose in providing information concerning statistical data, documentation of activities, follow-up evaluation, and reference needs. The records and reports commonly used in staff development are the master plan, the specific plans of the learning offerings, the annual report, interim report, individual employee and group records of attendance and achievement, statistical records, evaluations, budget records, and national or statewide standards." [14]

In summary, a brief discussion of the situational aspect of the nursing leadership process in nursing service and nursing inservice education has been presented. This process is part of the function of every professional nurse. The nurse will decide, relate, influence, and facilitate the behavior of peers, patients, and auxiliary and interdisciplinary personnel through communication to determine and achieve nursing service and institutional goals. Inservice education or staff development has been discussed as part of the answer to augment and strengthen the nursing leadership process. It is not a panacea that will solve nursing service problems, but when well-planned and well-executed, inservice education programs can help the nurse employee to develop and improve leadership behavior and thereby improve patient care in the health agency.

References

NURSING LEADERSHIP PROCESS IN NURSING EDUCATION

1. Miner J: Management Theory, Chap 2. New York, MacMillan Co, 1971.
2. Kazmier L: Principles of Management. New York, McGraw-Hill Book Co, 1960, pp 247-248.
3. Schein E: Process Consultation: Its Role in Organization Development. Reading, Mass, Addison-Wesley Pub Co, 1969.
4. Mosphet EL, Johns RL, Relles, TL: Educational Organization and Administration. Second edition. Englewood Cliffs, NJ, Prentice-Hall, 1967, pp 104-114.
5. McGregor D: The Human Side of Enterprise. New York, McGraw Hill Book Co, 1960.
6. Tannenbaum R, Schmidt HW: How to choose a leadership pattern. Harv Bus Rev 36:95-101, Mar-Apr 1958.
7. Herzberg F: Work and the Nature of Man. New York, World Publishing Company, 1966.
8. Mosphet EL, Johns RL, Relles, TL: Educational Organization and Administration. Second edition. Englewood Cliffs, NJ, Prentice-Hall, 1967, pp 107-110.

NURSING LEADERSHIP PROCESS IN NURSING SERVICE AND
INSERVICE EDUCATION

1. Schmidt WM: The professional nurse looks at her leadership responsibility, Leadership in Nursing Series: Looking into Nursing

Leadership, Executive Library, Washington, DC, Leadership Resources, Inc, 1966, p 1.
2. Hagen E, Wolff L: Nursing Leadership Behavior in General Hospitals. New York, Institute of Research and Service in Nursing Education, Teachers College, Columbia University, 1961, p 80.
3. *Idem:* p 81.
4. *Idem:* p 108.
5. *Idem:* p 109
6. *Idem:* p 147.
7. *Idem:* p 148.
8. Cooper SS, Hornback, MI: Continuing Nursing Education. New York, McGraw-Hill Book Co, 1973, p 175.
9. Tobin HM, Yoder PA, Hull PK, Scott BC: The Process of Staff Development, Component for Change. St. Louis, CV Mosby Company, 1974, pp 22-23.
10. American Nurses' Association: Statement of beliefs on inservice education and functions and qualifications for inservice educators. New York, American Nurses Association, 1966.
11. Magner MM: Inservice Education Manual for the Nursing Department. St. Louis, The Catholic Hospital Association, 1974, p 19.
12. Price EM: Learning Needs of Registered Nurses. New York, Teachers' College, Columbia University, 1967, p 52.
13. Eng E: Staff Development in a Hospital Nursing Service. New York, National League for Nursing, 1972, p 12.
14. Tobin HM, Yoder PA, Hull PK, Scott BC: The Process of Staff Development, Component for Change. St. Louis, CV Mosby Company, 1974, pp 22-23.

CHAPTER 6
Next Steps for Nursing Leadership

To fulfill its commitment to give nursing care to the sick and to help maintain the wellness of its citizens, nursing needs a plentiful supply of effective leaders. Nursing leaders are needed as practitioners, educators, administrators, researchers, theorists, and consultants.

The preceding chapters reviewed the state of leadership and nursing leadership today, focusing on theoretical formulations that are most applicable, and making some distinctions between and among concepts related to leadership. Efforts have been made to operationalize some of the best tenets found on leadership as proposed by thinkers, theorists, and researchers. It has been said that it takes 50 years for a good idea or good research results to take hold. We have attempted to close this gap—so that good ideas and research results are not held in abeyance while practitioners seek answers to questions and solutions to problems unmindful that these answers and solutions are already available. What is known remains academic achievement until utilized and operationalized in practice. It was necessary to fashion the available knowledge, choosing selectively,

Next Steps for Nursing Leadership   195

for use in the nursing situation—with its goals, expectations, and multiple public groups for interaction and service.

The next steps in nursing leadership are to test some of the ideas proposed in this text, especially as they relate to the nursing leadership process. Also needed is further operationalization of the leadership theory for nursing so that its goal in society can be fulfilled and it can maintain the autonomy it presently has and constantly needs. For leaders to make an impact on the health care system they must provide the services citizens need and they must be accountable for this service. Some mechanism, some way of making certain that the authority, influence, and power required to ensure that nursing fulfills its role are protected, developed, and rightfully used is needed.

Five steps have been delineated to further the development of nursing leadership:

Step 1. Define and designate what, when, where, and how the learning needed for the preparation of nurse leaders will be offered in baccalaureate, masters, and doctoral programs in nursing.

Inherent in this step is deliberate planning by nursing faculty members in these programs to designate the precise learnings, the place at which these learnings will take place, and the description of the teaching–learning strategies to ensure that behavioral expectations become a reality. Numerous learnings with behavioral counterparts needed to utilize the nursing leadership process were discussed in Chapter 4. Inherent is the need to keep leadership and nursing leadership behavioral expectations foremost in the curricular designs for baccalaureate, master, and doctoral degree programs in nursing. It is necessary to account for and facilitate the transfer of the general education and humanities base and the progressive liberal arts learnings in the baccalaureate, masters, and doctoral programs in nursing to be sure that the nursing process, the nursing leadership process, and the research process are learned.

Step 2. Seek to admit students who have the capacity to decide, to relate, to influence, and to facilitate the actions of others. Qualified students who have demonstrated leadership in elementary and high school and college should be sought.

Stogdill's survey of leadership research and the literature showed that persons who demonstrated leadership in elementary school, high school, and college would be likely to continue to demonstrate leadership throughout their adult lives.[1] Gardner made a plea for careful selectivity and admission of students when he said:

> This is particularly important for the segment of the population which is to exercise leadership in the society. If one is concerned to bring into the leadership ranks of a profession or a class or a society the men best qualified to exercise that leadership, the most sensible thing is to guard the door with rigorous selection procedures, rigorous procedures for testing ability, rigorous courses of preparation. And the purpose of the rigor is not simply to screen out the *less able* but to screen out the *less highly motivated.* The ones who get through will then be not only men of superior ability but men of superior character. The very fact of their surmounting difficult obstacles will have accomplished a vitally important sorting out.[2]

Thus, in addition to selecting students with the most potential to decide, to relate, to influence, and to facilitate, a history of experience as a leader must also be elected and recorded.

Step. 3. Foster the continuing development of theory applicable to the nursing process and to the nursing leadership process and support their applicability in all nursing practice settings.

Professional nursing practice is based on sound theory. There can be no practice without theory. This has been supported by theorists and practitioners alike and is receiving more support and more coverage in the literature. Hanlon and Thompson provide treatises in support of the belief that theory must guide practice.

> Since applied knowledge is by definition knowledge of the rules and procedures for the application of theory, then applied knowledge cannot be given where theoretical knowledge does not exist. . . . If a person does not have knowledge of the nature, purpose, structure, and function of the

work he is to perform, then we cannot give him true applied knowledge. What we can do—and often actually do—is to supply the person with 'cookbook' or 'how to do it' knowledge. In that case, the person is a technician. He may be a skilled worker. Most certainly he is not a professional. He does not know what he is doing and why he is doing it at every stage of the work.[3]

Thompson, an educator, concurs with this view when she says education (nursing, too), like any systematic endeavor,

. . . needs an overall strategy—a collection of systematically related concepts which accounts for its endeavors. Such a directive role is the function of theory. Theories are not just vague, whispy musings. Theories are the guideposts which hold together and direct our undertakings. . . . A theory is intended to be the skeletal structure which, when fleshed out by either research or practice, becomes the guide which spawns new knowledge and improved practice.[4]

Step 4. Design research studies to test the validity of the nursing leadership process and the specific application of leadership theory to the nursing situation.

No profession can exist without research to develop its body of knowledge and to test its strategies to insure that its actions make a difference. Research is the mainstay for nursing —for testing theories and for validating nursing actions. The nursing process and the nursing leadership process should be researched. In addition, the data comprising these processes as well as the nursing strategies originating from judgments about the data applied to resolve client problems should be tested.

Step 5. Support continuing education for nursing leaders, potential nurse leaders, and particularly, for persons expected to be leaders but who are unprepared for strategic positions in nursing.

Nurses prepared in baccalaureate, masters, and doctoral programs in nursing are part of the community of scholars, where the purpose is to prepare an educated person as well as a professional nursing practitioner—generalist and specialist. Nurses are prepared to be learners for life. No one need tell the professional nursing practitioner that she needs to keep up to date; she knows this. Built into the triad of processes utilized for nursing, is the evaluation of one's thoughts and actions. The professional nursing practitioner readily knows her strengths, her limitations, and the effort and direction needed to offset her limitations.

Further, the professional nursing practitioner should select career opportunities for which she is prepared or for which she has the basic preparation, but with study, time, and practice will manage and meet the demands of the situation. Multiple means and sources are available for continuing education. More than anyone else, the nurse leader should know what, when, how and why continuing education is a must for herself.

In conclusion, nurse leaders can be prepared *deliberately* in the numbers needed to ensure citizens the best nursing service from the most appropriately prepared nursing practitioners at the time it is needed for well or ill persons wherever they are. Mastery of the nursing leadership process, the nursing process, and the research process with a firm background knowledge of supporting theories constitute the triad of processes synonymous with nursing leadership.

Our final message for the nurse leader is:

Do not follow where the path may lead. Go instead where there is no path and leave a trail.

References

1. Stogdill R: Handbook of Leadership. New York, Free Press, 1974, p 176.
2. Gardner JW: Excellence. New York, Harper & Row Publishers, 1961, p 100.
3. Hanlon J: Theory and practice of nursing. J Contin Educ Nurs 5:15, Nov-Dec 1974.
4. Thompson LJ: The nature and need of theory. Educ Forum 39:474, 1975.

Appendix

OPINIONNAIRE

Introduction

Exploration of ideas about nursing leadership has produced some interesting results. To corroborate or refute our ideas, we invite your participation and ask you to respond to the items recorded on these two pages. Assuming your willingness to participate, we express our gratitude to you and we assure you that names of participant's will not be disclosed.

Thank you

Part I

1. Define the following terms: (alphabetical listing)
   Administration
   Leadership
   Management
   Supervision
2. List the actions you perceive as essential to each.

Administration	Leadership	Management	Supervision

3. Number each of these four terms in order of priority as you perceive them; identify the most inclusive as No. 1, and enumerate the remaining three in descending order.
4. Comments:

Part II

1. Indicate whether and why you agree or disagree with each of the following definitions:

a. **Nursing leadership** is a process whereby a person who is a nurse effects the actions of others in goal determination and goal achievement.
Agree ( )   Disagree ( )
Reason(s) for response:

b. **Nursing leadership process** is the means by which determined goals are achieved through the actions of deciding, relating, influencing and facilitating.
Agree ( )   Disagree ( )
Reason(s) for response:

2. The following are four actions identified as inherent in the nursing leadership process:

        Deciding
        Relating
        Influencing
        Facilitating

Do you perceive these actions as essential to the nursing leadership process?
Agree ( )   Disagree ( )
Reason(s) for response:

3. Place these terms in order of priority as you perceive them; identify the most essential as No. 1, next as No. 2, etc:

    1. _____
    2. _____
    3. _____
    4. _____

INTRODUCTION

A group of 125 students, enrolled in the School of Nursing at The Catholic University of America, agreed to respond to a request for opinions. Twenty-one students were seniors in the baccalaureate nursing program, while 95 were in the first semester and 9 in the fourth and last semester of the masters program. Analysis of the 125 responses reveals that the four terms: administration, leadership, management, and supervision, lack clarity. This lack applies to the baccalaureate as well as to the masters' candidates. Some used terms to define management similar to the terms others used to define administration. Some could find no differences between the terms administration, management, and supervision. A few mentioned that leadership permeates and applies to each of these three terms. Leadership was the only one of the four terms defined in a somewhat different way by many of the respondents. Even though none of the four terms could be defined precisely, certain generalities, certain trends evolved as the definitions of the terms suggested by respondents were studied.

Definition of Administration, Leadership, Management, and Supervision

BACCALAUREATE SENIOR STUDENTS

The baccalaureate groups ($N = 21$) perceived *administration* as that group of persons who are recognized as the leaders of an organization; this means they are the top of the hierarchy, the overseers, the head of the total, entire, or whole agency. Hence, the focus is on the overall, not on specifics. These persons are the governing force of the organization and have control. They are responsible for:

(a) Maintaining the integrity and function of the total agency so that maximum potential can be realized.
(b) Setting rules, priorities, values, policies, boundaries, limitations, guidelines, procedures, and goals and communicating these to appropriate persons.
(c) Certain tasks, such as raising funds, planning activities, and necessary paper work, that enable the agency to exist and perpetuate itself.
(d) Providing an environment conducive to efficient functioning and through the coordination of group efforts encourage smooth and harmonious functioning so that goals can be accomplished.
(e) Liaison activities between the organization and the community.

Their perception of *leadership* suggests that this is a personal attribute, one that involves some authority and communicates certain qualities and responsibilities, namely:

The quality of being:

(a) innovative; able to initiate new ideas;
(b) self-confident;
(c) a change agent;
(d) able to set high ideals;
(e) able to constructively use education and experience in coping with new or stressful situations;
(f) able to think positively.

The responsibilities of leadership include:

(a) helping others obtain a common goal;
(b) directing the activities of the group;
(c) being accountable for prescribed actions;
(d) performing according to certain established standards;
(e) keeping abreast of current happenings;
(f) commending work well done;
(g) accomplishing goals;
(h) promoting group equilibrium;
(i) motivating others;
(j) following as well as giving directions.

Leadership is viewed with a very personal flavor in which there is group involvement, with certain expectations of the person or persons who will direct the group toward its purpose. In order to realize anticipated outcomes, however, the persons endowed with such potential need to occupy a position where such abilities can be used.

Most of the baccalaureate group perceive *management* as an action-oriented term. These views are represented by defining management using phrases such as the following:

(a) Body of people who deal with practicality; they decide how policy decisions will be carried out, how values and policies will be defined, how priorities and goals will be set.
(b) People who carry out the activities of the group; they carry out the plans and do the physical work required.
(c) Essentially this group handles the everday "hassles," keep things rolling.

Other factors identified as inherent in management include:

(a) Control—being in control of a group;
—being in charge of an area.
(b) Responsibility—for the persons involved in a situation;
—for the smooth running of an operation;
—for getting a job done correctly;
—for establishing proper priorities;
—for planning and organizing activities;
—for the manner in which actions are performed.
(c) Guidance—of the functioning of a business;
—of the people who are functioning.
(d) Coordinating—work hours;
—staffing;
—financial activities;
—the functions of the group.
(e) Delegation—of responsibilities according to the abilities of the workers and the needs of the consumers;
—to ensure effective use of manpower.

Certain components of management identified by the baccalaureate group were rather unique and individual.

Management is:

(a) the use of skills which are on a rather dictatorial level, not democratic;
(b) secondary to administration and supervision;
(c) a corporate structure as opposed to labor;
(d) the participation with other workers and being able to perform the same technical skills, but possessing leadership which elevates one to the management position;
(e) representing the owners;
(f) the boss—has nothing to do with leadership abilities.

Supervision is defined by the baccalaureate group as:

direct governing of subgroups of subordinates;
dealing more with "people" and of running a business;
overseeing responsibilities for actions and functions of a group of people;

Appendix 205

no direct participation except when needed in cases of indecision or error;
suggesting alternatives;
maintaining order and maximum function;
overseeing own and others work to ensure correct completion and in proper order;
direction in any situation;
"more select group of people to keep in line";
main guide to a particular group;
synonymous with management but singular in essence;
liaison between administration and those supervised, and planners;
ensure environment for practitioner;
offer support, counsel, instruction;
oversee operation of institution or group;
running according to plan;
availability of resource persons to advise on departmental problems;
observation and evaluation by experienced able person over another person or group less qualified;
resource person for a group;
observer of actions, support of workers who are knowledgeable in field;
overseers of actions; coordinators, close and helpful guidance of others;
keeping check over others to see that job is done; independent role of guidance, support and assistance; assessment by person(s) of the produced efforts of others to determine quality of performance and suitable job assignment for that person.

2. MASTERS, FIRST-YEAR STUDENTS

These 95 respondents see *administration* as a broad activity of persons who are at the top level of an organization; some speak of levels, some refer to hierarchy, and all perceive steps or progressive phases in the four terms.

The "broad activities" are those policy-making functions, which include determining policy, enforcing policy, and/or making policy. Each of these presents a different role of the person in administration.

"Control" is a word frequently used to define administration; "the body who exercises and/or maintains total control"; the group with the "controlling power."

Responsibility and authority are characteristic of this group; they are the "backbone of the organization," should see that the "operation runs smoothly," should formulate guidelines, and provide overall coordination of activities. They are responsible for making major decisions.

An additional facet of the administrative role was identified as financing and budgeting. As ones on the top echelon, the person-oriented tasks are identified as well as the nonperson-oriented tasks dealing with money, budget, financial, and legal matters. One respondent summed up the definition by stating that administration is "the big boss."

Leadership was viewed by the 91 respondents as "the art of persuading someone to do something he does not want to do." Several suggest that leadership is a learned role, a learned capability that involves the use of certain powers that are necessary to lead a group in a joint endeavor.

The role of the leaders was seen as motivating others, inspiring others, directing the actions of others, influencing others, teaching others, acting as role model for others.

Leadership suggests that the leader has enough knowledge to be self-confident in his position so that responsible decisions can be reached, good interpersonal relations can be maintained, and that the leader is open to the risks involved in change. Originality, creativity, and initiative were all mentioned as essential features of leadership. One person suggested that the leader is distinguished by possession of charismatic qualities.

The first-year masters students defined *management* in a more technical way. They suggest that management is the "efficient" level between administration and the "grass roots." Managers carry out policies set by others and therefore have no opportunity for innovation. They are concerned with getting a job done in the most economic way. Although a few respondents perceive management as a decision making body responsible for carrying out the goals of administration, others see the manager as a "subdivision of administration," as the ones who coordinate business matters, as the ones who keep everything in harmony, the ones who lead the group toward a goal.

The 95 graduate student respondents describe the *supervisor's* role as guiding, directing, assisting others, and acting as a role model and resource person. The supervisor accomplishes tasks usually through other persons. Overseeing the activities of others, especially for the purpose of judging their accomplishments, is an activity of the supervisor. Responsibility for establishing standards that provide a base for evaluation was mentioned by a few; these characteristics are similar to others dealing with intervention activities, as needed for teaching, and day-to-day attention to quality and quantity of services being performed. Some respondents saw supervisors providing an atmosphere conducive to communication, and the sharing of ideas and goals.

3. Masters, Second-Year Students

The 9 respondents enrolled in the second year of the masters program saw *administration* as a broad, rather than a specific level of functioning. One-third of the group felt that administration involves being responsible for coordinating and organizing the work tasks of the total unit; administration also involves directing the actions of others, goal planning, and guiding the actions of the group.

Leadership is perceived as exerting influence on others so that goals can be accomplished. The leader does this by acting as a role model, by being creative, by providing initiative and needed resources, by directing and guiding others in the problem-solving process. One person suggested that leadership is "an individual human quality unique to (a few) persons."

Management is seen by these 9 persons as operating on a more specific level than does administration. The person functioning in management sets up guidelines, defines goals, does the mechanical work necessary to keep action progressing, defines and directs the actions of others.

Supervision does not "necessarily involve leadership." Persons who supervise are responsible for smaller groups of persons, they serve as liaison between administration and persons on lower levels in an organization; besides directing the activities of others, the supervisor helps employees identify strengths and weaknesses so that strengths can be enhanced and weaknesses improved.

Summary and Comments

Many activities were identified in all four areas; for example, assessing, planning, and evaluating were mentioned as important in all four areas of functioning. A few specific activities were identified in only one area to make it more distinct from the others; for example, research was identified in administration and in leadership, but not in management and supervision. Managing was labeled as an activity under supervision and administration and leadership; supervision was an activity included under managing and leadership. Only under leadership did actions of role model, creativity, and initiative appear. One person suggested that "guts" was a quality of leadership. Both management and supervision included actions that are more technically or task oriented.

The comments from this group of respondents suggest that without leadership, one cannot be successful in the other areas. Leadership seems to permeate all areas of functioning and should do so. However, to more carefully delineate the unique aspects of each of the terms, additional research is needed.

The respondents were asked to identify actions they perceived as essential to each of the four terms: administration, leadership, management, and supervision. Essentially, the actions that were listed were the same actions (by terminology and by influence) as those identified in the definitions of each term. No unique actions were identified in this section.

Order of Priority Defined by Respondents to Four Terms: Leaderships, Administration, Management, and Supervision.
(Not all respondents completed each section of the opinionnaire.)

1. BACCALAUREATE SENIOR STUDENTS
   $N = 21$

	L	A	M	S
1	18	2	0	1
2	1	9	6	5
3	2	4	10	5
4	0	6	5	10

2. MASTERS, FIRST-YEAR STUDENTS
   N = 54

	L	A	M	S
1	38	12	2	2
2	3	22	18	11
3	4	8	22	20
4	9	22	12	21

3. MASTERS, SECOND-YEAR STUDENTS
   N = 9

	L	A	M	S
1	6	3	1	0
2	0	3	4	2
3	1	3	2	3
4	2	0	2	4

Definition of Nursing Leadership

The group of students were asked to respond to three items:

(a) whether and why they agree or disagree with the definition of nursing leadership;
(b) whether and why they agree or disagree with the definition of nursing leadership process;
(c) whether and why they agree or disagree with the four actions of deciding, relating, influencing, and facilitating being essential to the nursing leadership process.

1. BACCALAUREATE SENIOR STUDENTS

Nineteen persons agreed with the definition of nursing leadership. Five gave no reason for agreeing. For those 14 who gave reasons, their comments mainly reiterated the thoughts contained in the printed definition. One person emphasized that leaders must be pace-setters and provide examples, i.e., be role models.

Of the two who disagreed, one felt the definition does not clearly identify the nurse's involvement in leadership; another felt that a leader does not have a right to determine the goals of another person.

2. MASTERS, FIRST-YEAR STUDENTS

Ten of 94 respondents indicated that they disagreed with the definition of leadership. Two questioned the word: "effects" and felt that "affects" would be a more appropriate description of what the nurse does. One felt that the nurse must also be instrumental in "initiating goals of her own" as well as be concerned with the goals of others. One person disagreed without stating a reason.

Three objected to the use of the word "nurse" in the definition stating that "this is not to say that it is not better for nurses to lead nurses, but simply that it is too narrow to be exclusive." Nursing leadership doesn't necessarily have to "come from a person who is a nurse."

One person suggested that "nurses are not usually considered leaders." The implication was, however, that depending upon "level of education, individual initiative, and creativity," a nurse may be a leader. One person suggested that only the individual himself can set his own personal goals, apparently objecting to the idea that nurses have a responsibility to help others set their goals.

One respondent felt that a nurse could affect the actions of others in a negative way, so the definition should suggest a positive influence and a progression desirable to make the definition more acceptable.

Fifteen of the 94 respondents agreed with the definition but gone no reason for their response.

Six persons agreed with the definition but stated conditions of agreement or that they agreed partially with the definition. Suggestions for inclusion in the definition were: allow for the idea that others in the group assist in goal setting and in defining how goals are to be achieved; ensure the effect the nurse has is a positive one; this is too narrow a definition; "nursing leadership encompasses much more"; the leader "does not have to be a nurse."

The remainder (63) of the 94 respondents agreed with the definition and amplified upon the printed definition in a variety of ways and by using a number of synonyms. Many merely reiterated certain phrases for emphasis.

3. MASTERS, SECOND-YEAR STUDENTS:

Eight of this group agreed with the definition of nursing leadership. One disagreed, because, she reasoned, the word "effects" is ambiguous; it allows for the interpretation that the nurse can "effect" other's actions in a negative way; that is, may hinder the movement of the group toward the defined goal. The interpretation of the word "effects" in this manner is contrary to the respondents' view of leadership, which has an implied positive quality or aspect.

Eight students agreed because:

leadership is involved with goal setting; and determining how and by whom goals will be met;
leadership involves influencing and motivating actions more than controlling actions;
this is how nursing leadership has been perceived;
the nurse affects the actions of others only by assisting via suggestions and/or recommendations as requested by the person who is defining his goals;
providing leadership implies responsibility for setting guidelines for others.

Definitions of Nursing Leadership Process

1. BACCALAUREATE SENIOR STUDENTS

Nineteen agreed with the definition of nursing leadership process. Seven of the 19 gave no reason. Of the 12 who stated reasons, most reiterated the elements of the definitions by using synonyms and manipulating the printed words to be consistent with their own style of speaking or writing. Some merely said: "good"; "sounds good"; "it's logical"; "sums up my feelings."

Two disagreed with the definition; one did not like the word "facilitating" and one wished to add communication and evaluating to the actions.

2. MASTERS, FIRST-YEAR STUDENTS

Ninety of the respondents agreed with the definition of nursing leadership process.

Of the 59 reasons stated for agreeing with the definition; several suggested it follows a logical sequence of actions, is related to the nursing process, as it should be.

One stated that without these aspects, there is neither a process nor leadership. Communication was suggested as a necessary ingredient.

Seven of these 59 persons raised some questions about the definition being too broad, whether these actions would be considered deliberate or conscious on the part of the leaders. It was also suggested that this definition implies the leader has all the answers, which is unrealistic. Another suggestion was to include a feedback mechanism to provide for the evaluation of leader as well as followers.

Thrity-one persons agreed with the definition without stating a reason. Three persons disagreed because the definition was not specific enough and evaluative aspects were not adequately identified. One person was not sure whether to agree or disagree because the terms were too difficult to differentiate.

3. MASTERS, SECOND-YEAR STUDENTS

Eight persons agreed with the definitions of nursing leadership process. Comments included the condition that the idea of evaluation was included in the actions of deciding and relating; one stressed that when positive actions are viewed as relevant, the process of leadership is facilitated and the ones being influenced are stimulated through motivation and explanation to follow the example of the leader. Two persons felt this is the most realistic way, the most democratic, and the most essential way to accomplish aims; one person suggested that the action of teaching should be incorporated in the definition.

One person disagreed with the definition because she perceived two essentials omitted—elements of communication (individual and/or group), and data analysis to develop strategies of action.

All 9 agreed these four actions are essential to the nursing leadership process. Cited as reasons for their agreement were ideas that today, nursing is dependent on good relations with others and upon successfully influencing those with whom relations must be established; these actions are essential to the problem-solving process, to the goal setting process, to the achievement of quality care; the interdependence of these actions enhance the group leader's role.

Actions Inherent in the Nursing Leadership Process

The respondents who commented about these actions redefined and restated elements of the definitions they had previously cited. Analysis of the responses provided no additional data.

Order of Priority Defined by Respondents for Four Actions— Deciding, Relating, Influencing, and Facilitating
(not all respondents completed each section of the opinionnaire).

1. BACCALAUREATE SENIOR STUDENTS
   $N = 20$

	D	R	I	F
1	10	9	1	0
2	7	7	4	2
3	1	2	10	7
4	2	2	5	11

2. MASTERS, FIRST-YEAR STUDENTS
   $N = 91$

	D	R	I	F
1	32	36	10	13
2	21	35	20	15
3	17	14	39	21
4	21	6	22	42

3. MASTERS, SECOND-YEAR STUDENTS
   $N = 9$

	D	R	I	F
1	4	2	2	1
2	1	5	1	2
3	3	0	2	4
4	1	2	4	2

BIBLIOGRAPHY

Abdellah F: Criterion measures in nursing. Nurs Res 10:21-26, 1961. pp 21-26.

Abrahamson M: The Professional in the Organization. Chicago, Rand McNally, 1967.

Aiken L, Aiken J: A systematic approach to the evaluation of interpersonal relationships. Am J Nurs 73:863-867, 1973.

Aiken M, Mott P(eds): The Structure of Community Power. New York, Random House, 1970.

Aikens C: Hospital Training-School Methods and the Head Nurse. Philadelphia, WB Saunders Co, 1914.

Alexander E: Nursing Administration in the Hospital Care System. St. Louis, CV Mosby, 1972.

Alford RR, Scoble HM: Community leadership, education, and political behavior. Am Sociol Rev 33:259-272, 1968.

American Nurses' Association: Facts About Nursing, 1973-1974. Kansas City, American Nurses Association, 1974.

American Nurses' Association: Standards for Nursing Services. Kansas City, Mo, American Nurses' Association, 1973.

American Nurses Foundation: International Directory of Nurses with Doctoral Degrees. Kansas City, American Nurses Foundation, Inc, 1973.

Anderson LR: Leader behavior, member attitudes, and task performance of intercultural discussion groups. J Sociol Psychol 69:305-319, 1966.

Anderson LR, Fiedler FE: The effect of participatory and supervisory leadership on group creativity. J Appl Psychol 48:277-236, 1964.

Anderson R: Activity preferences and leadership behavior of head nurses. Nurs Res Part I 13:239-243, Summer 1964; Part II 13:333-337, Fall 1964.

Argyris C: Integrating the Individual and the Organization. New York, John Wiley and Sons, 1964.

Argyris C: Interpersonal Competence and Organizational Effectiveness. Homewood, Illinois, Irwin-Dorsey, 1962.

Argyris C: Management and Organizational Development. New York, McGraw-Hill Book Co, 1971.

Argyris C: Organizational leadership, Leadership and Interpersonal Behavior. Edited by L Petrullo, BM Bass. New York, Holt, Rinehart and Winston, 1961.

Arndt C, Hucksbay L: Nursing Administration: Theory for Practice with a Systems Approach. St. Louis, CV Mosby Co, 1975.

Ashley JA: This I believe about power in nursing. Nurs Outlook 21:637-641, 1973.

Association for Supervision and Curriculum Development: Yearbook 1960: Leadership for Improvement of Instruction. Washington, National Education Association, 1960.

Bailey J, Claus K: Decision Making in Nursing. St. Louis, CV Mosby Co, 1975.

Baldridge JV(ed): Academic Governance. Berkeley, Calif, McCutchen Publishers, 1971.

Baldridge JV: Power and Conflict in the University. New York, John Wiley and Sons, 1971.

Banathy B: Instructional Systems. Palo Alto, Calif, Fearon Publishers, 1968.

Barber JD: Power in Communities: An Experiment in the Governmental Process. Chicago, Rand McNally, 1966.

Barnard C: The Functions of the Executive. Cambridge, Mass, Harvard University Press, 1964.

Bartlett CJ: Dimensions of leadership behavior in classroom discussion groups. J Educ Psychol 50:280-284, 1959.

Bass BM: Leadership, Psychology, and Organizational Behavior. New York, Harper, 1960.

Bates B, Chamberlin RW: Physician leadership as perceived by nurses. Nurs Res 19:534-539, 1970.

Bauer R: The obstinate audience: the influence process from the point of view of social communication. Am Psychologist 19:319-328, 1964.

Baumgartel H: Leadership styles as a variable in research administration. Admin Sci Q 2:344-360, 1957.

Bavelas A: Leadership: man and function. Admin Sci Q 4:491-498, 1960.

Bell W, Hill R, Wright C: Public Leadership. San Francisco, Chandler Publishing Co, 1961.

Bellows RM: Creative Leadership. Englewood Cliffs, NJ, Prentice-Hall, 1959.

Bennis W: Changing Organizations. New York. McGraw-Hill Book Co, 1966.

Bennis W, Benne K, Chin R(eds): The Planning of Change. New York, Holt, Rinehart and Winston, 1961.

Bennis WG: Leadership theory and administrative behavior: the problems of authority. Admin Sci Q 5:259-301, 1959.

Bennis WG, Berkowitz N, Affinito M, Malone M: Authority, power and the ability to influence. Hum Relat 11:143-155, 1958.

Benson H: Your innate asset for combating stress. Harv Bus Rev 52:49-60, July-Aug 1974.

Berg IA, Bass BM: Conformity and Deviation. New York, Harper, 1961.

Bevelas A: Leadership: man and function. Admin Sci Q 4:491-498, 1960.

Beyers M, Phillpis C: Nursing Management for Patient Care. Boston, Little, Brown and Co, 1971.

Bhushan LI: A scale of leadership preference. Psychol Studies 14:28-34, 1969.
Biddle BJ, Thomas EJ: Role Theory: Concepts and Research. New York, John Wiley and Sons, 1966.
Bierstedt R: An analysis of social power. Am Sociol Rev 15:730-736, 1950.
Biggs DA, Huneryager SG, Delaney JJ: Leadership behavior: interpersonal needs and effective supervisory training. Personnel Psychol 19:311-320, 1966.
Blau P: Exchange and Power in Social Life. New York, John Wiley and Sons, 1964.
Blau P: On the Nature of Organizations. New York, John Wiley and Sons, 1974.
Blau P: The hierarchy of authority in organizations. Am J Sociol 73:453-467, 1968.
Blau P: The Organization of Academic Work. New York, John Wiley and Sons, 1973.
Bloom B(ed): Taxonomy of Educational Objectives: The Classification of Educational Goals. Handbook I: Cognitive Domain. New York, David McKay Co, 1956.
Bloom M: The Paradox of Helping. New York, John Wiley and Sons, 1975.
Bloom MT: The great communications dilemma. J Nurs Admin 1(6): 29-34, 1971.
Bonjean CM: Class, status, and power reputation. Sociol Soc Res 49:69-75, 1964.
Bonjean CM: Community leadership: a case study and conceptual refinement. Am J Sociol 67:672-681, 1963.
Bowman R, Culpepper R: Power: Rx for change. Am J Nurs 74:1053-1056, 1974.
Brennan WJ, Cole ME: Meeting demands for change. Hospitals 45(17): 65-67, 1971.
Bridges EM, Doyle WF, Mahan DF: Effects of hierarchical differentiation on group productivity, efficiency, and risk taking. Admin Sci Q 13:305-319, 1968.
Bross ID: Design for Decision. New York, MacMillan Co, 1953.
Brothers J: The woman as boss. Mainliner, Mar 1974, pp 32-35, 57.
Brown JS: Risk, propensity in decision making: a comparison of business and public school administrators. Admin Sci Q 15:473-481, 1970.
Brown AF: Reactions to leadership. Educ Admin Q 3:62-73, 1967.
Burnstein E: An analysis of group decision involving risk ("the risky shift"). Hum Relat 22:381-395, 1969.
Cartwright D: Achieving change in people: some applications of group dynamics theory. Hum Rel 4(4):381, 1951.

Cartwright D: Influence, leadership control, Handbook of Organizations. Edited by JB March. Chicago, Rand McNally, 1965, pp 1-57.

Cartwright D, Zander A(eds): Group Dynamics: Research and Theory. Third edition. New York, Harper & Row Publishers, 1968.

Christman L: Nursing leadership—style and substance. Am J Nurs 67: 2091-2093, 1967.

Clark B: Faculty organization and authority, Academic Governance. Edited by JV Baldridge. Berkeley, Calif, McCutchan Publishers, 1971, pp 236-249.

Cleveland H: How do you get everybody in on the act and still get some action. Educ Record, Summer 1974, pp 177-182.

Cleveland H, Lasswell H: Ethics and Bigness. New York, Harper and Brothers, 1962.

Clissold G, Metz E: Evaluation—a tangible process. Nurs Outlook 14:41-45, March 1966.

Cochan TC, Ransen P: Developing an evaluation tool by group action. Am J Nurs 62:94-97, Mar 1962.

Collier A: Management, Men, and Values. New York, Harper & Row Publishers, 1962.

Combs A, Avila D, Purkey W: Helping Relationships, Basic Concepts for the Helping Professions. Boston, Allyn and Bacon Inc, 1971.

Condon Sr MB, Johnain C, Oliver B: An experience in change. J Cont Ed Nurs 6(6):2-16, 1975.

Conference on Preparation for Leadership in Psychiatric Nursing Service. New York, Department of Nursing Education, Teachers College, Columbia University, June 7-8, 1963.

Conley A: Instructional leadership in curriculum development in baccalaureate programs in nursing. New York, Columbia University 1972. Abstracted in Disser Abs Int 33:2610-a, Dec 1972.

Cussler M: The Woman Executive. New York, Harcourt Brace and World, 1958.

Dalton G, Barnes L, Zaleznik A: The Distribution of Authority in Formal Organization. Cambridge, MIT Press, 1968.

Department of Health, Education, and Welfare: Extending the Scope of Nursing Practice. Report of Secretary's Committee to Study Extended Roles for Nurses. Washington, US Government Printing Office, 1971.

Dibden A(ed): The Academic Deanship in American Colleges and Universities. Carbondale, Ill, Southern Illinois University Press, 1968.

Diers D: Leadership problems and possibilities in nursing. Am J Nurs, 72:1447, 1972.

Dietrich B, Miller D: Nursing leadership—a theoretical framework. Nurs Outlook 14:52-55, Aug 1966.

Division of Nursing: Planning for Nursing Needs and Resources. Be-

thesda, Maryland, US Department of Health, Education, and Welfare, Division of Nursing, Apr 1972.
Donnelly P: A philosophy of change. Hosp Prog 44:71-74, 1963, pp 71-74.
Donovan HM: Toward an understanding of leadership and supervision. Superv Nurs 3:22-24, Oct 1972.
Douglass L, Bevis O: Nursing Leadership in Action. Second edition. St. Louis, CV Mosby Co, 1974.
Downton J: Rebel Leadership. New York, Free Press, 1973.
Drucker P: The Effective Executive. New York, Harper & Row Publishers, 1966.
Drucker P: Technology, Management, and Society. New York, Harper & Row Publishers, 1970.
Dubno P: Leadership, group effectiveness, and speed of decision. J Soc Psychol 65:351-360, 1965.
Duncan J: The curriclum director in curriculum change. Educ Forum 38:51-76, Nov 1973.
Durbin R, Springall W: Organization and Administration of Health Care. St. Louis, CV Mosby Co, 1969.
Eggers ET: The essence of leadership. Superv Nurse 3, 23-27, Dec 1972.
Elsberry NL: Power relations in hospital nursing. J Nurs Adm 2(5):75-77, Sept-Oct 1972.
Emmet D: Rules, Roles, and Relations. New York, St. Martin's Press, 1966.
Etzioni A: Organization control structure, Handbook of Organizations. Edited by J March. Chicago, Rand-McNally, 1965, pp 652-677.
Etzioni A: The Semi-professions and Their Organization. New York, The Free Press, 1969.
Farris GF, Lim FG: Effects of performance on leadership, cohesiveness, influence, satisfaction, and subsequent performance. J Appl Psychol 53:490-497, 1969.
Feshel A. Pottker J: Women in educational governance: a statistical portrait. Educ Researcher 3:4-7, July-Aug 1974.
Fiedler FE: A Theory of Leadership Effectiveness. New York, McGraw-Hill Book Co, 1967.
Fiedler FE: Leadership. New York, General Learning Press, 1971.
Fiedler FE: The effects of leadership training and experience: a contingency model interpretation. Admin Sci Q 17:453-470, 1972.
Filley AC, Grimes AJ: The bases of power in decision processes. Proc Acad Mgmt, 1967.
Finer H: Administration and the Nursing Services. New York, The Macmillan Company, 1952.

Fleishman EA: Manual for Leadership Opinion Questionnaire. Chicago, Ill, Science Research Associate, 1969.

Flory C(ed): Managers for Tomorrow. New York, New American Library, Inc, 1965.

Fox D, Kelly R: The Research Process in Nursing. New York, Appleton-Century-Crofts, 1967.

French W: Personnel Management Process: Human Resources Administration. Second edition. Boston, Houghton Mifflin Co, 1970.

French JP, Snyder R: Leadership and interpersonal power, Studies in Social Power. Edited by D Cartwright. Ann Arbor, University of Michigan, Institute for Social Research, 1959.

Gage NL(ed): Handbook of Research on Teaching: A Project of the American Research Assoc. Chicago, Rand McNally, 1963.

Gagne R: Perspectives of Curriculum Evaluation. Chicago, Rand McNally, 1967.

Gamson W: Violence and political power: the meek don't make it. Psychol Today 8:35-41, July 1974.

Gardner J: The antileadership vaccine. Carnegie Corp of NY Annual Report. New York, 1965, pp 3-12.

Gardner J: Self-renewal. New York, Harper & Row Publishers, Inc, 1963.

Gardner J: No Easy Victories. New York, Harper & Row Publishers, Inc, 1968.

Gaspard NJ: Director of nursing in a comprehensive health center. Nurs Outlook 19:590-591, Sept 1971.

Gibbs CA: Leadership. In Lindzey A, Aronson E: The Handbook of Social Psychology. Vol 4, Second edition. Reading, Mass, Addison-Wesley Publishing Co, 1969.

Gibbs CA: The principles and traits of leadership, Leadership, Edited by CA Gibbs. Baltimore, Penguin Books, pp 205-213.

Gibbs CA(ed): Leadership: Selected Readings. Baltimore, Penguin Books, 1969.

Gibson JL: Organizational theory and the nature of man. J Acad Manag 19:233-245, 1966.

Gilbert MA: Personality profiles and leadership potential of medical-surgical and psychiatric nursing graduate students. Nurs Res 24:125-130, Mar-Apr 1975.

Gill W: Key concepts in management in nursing. Superv Nurse 20:21-28, February 1971.

Glaser W: Nursing Leadership and Policy: Some Cross-national Comparisons, The Nursing Profession. Edited by F Davis. New York, John Wiley and Sons, 1966.

Goble F: Excellence in Leadership. New York, American Management Association, 1972.

Goldstein AP, Sorcher M: Changing Supervisor Behavior. New York, Pergamon Press, Inc, 1974.
Golembiewski R: Men, Management, and Morality. New York, McGraw-Hill Book Co, 1965.
Golembiewski RT: Organizing Men and Power. Chicago, Rand McNally, 1967.
Goodstadt B, Kipnes D: Situational influences on the use of power. J Appl Psychol 54:201-207, 1970.
Gorham W: Methods of measuring staff nursing personnel. Nurs Res 12:4-11, Winter 1963.
Gould JW: The Academic Deanship. New York, Teachers College Press, Teachers College, Columbia University, 1967.
Graves H: Can nursing shed bureaucracy? Am J Nurs 71:491-494, Mar 1971.
Greenwood WT: Management and Organizational Behavioral Theories: An Interdisciplinary Approach. Cincinnati, South-Western Publishing Co, 1965.
Griffiths D: Administrative Theory. New York, Appleton-Century-Crofts, 1959.
Griffiths D(ed): Developing Taxonomies of Organizational Behavior in Education Administration. Chicago, Rand-McNally and Co, 1969.
Gruenfeld L and Kassum S: Supervisory style and organizational effectiveness in a pediatric hospital. Personnel Psychology, 26:531-544, Winter 1973.
Guan, HK: Creative leadership in supervision: the effects on students' behavior and performance. Nurs J Singapore 12:99-101, November 1972, abstracted in Nurs Res 22:363, July-Aug 1973.
Guerin QW: A functional approach to attitude change. Manag Rev 59(8): 33, 1970.
Guetzkow H, Forehand GA, James BJ: An evaluation of educational influence on administrative judgement. Admin Sci Q 6:483-500, 1962.
Gusfield JR: Functional areas of leadership in social movements. Sociol Q 7:137-156, 1966.
Haase P, Smith M: Nursing Education in the South 1973. Atlanta, Southern Regional Education Board, 1973.
Hagen E, Wolff L: Nursing Leadership Behavior in General Hospitals. New York, Teachers College, Columbia University, Institute of Research and Service in Nursing Education, 1961.
Hall B, Little D: Group project and learning outcomes. Nurs Outlook 17:82-83, June 1969.
Hall C: Who controls the nursing profession? Nurs Times 69: Suppl:89-92, June 7, 1973.
Hall, D, Nougaim K: An examination of Maslow's need hierarchy in an

organizational setting, organizational behavior and human performance. Nurs Outlook 16:12-16, Mar 1968.

Halpin AW: The behavior of leaders. Educ Leadership 14:172-176, 1956.

Hanlon J: Theory and practice of nursing. J Contin Educ Nurs 5:12-18, Nov-Dec 1974.

Harrison R: Understanding your organization's character. Harv Bus Rev 50(3):119-128, 1972.

Hawley W, Wirt F: The Search for Community Power. Englewood Cliffs, NJ, Prentice-Hall, 1968.

Hayes J: Criteria for managerial performance. Am Assembly Collegiate Schools Bus Bull 10(1):17-21, 1973.

Hemphill JK: Why people attempt to lead, Leadership and Interpersonal Behavior. Edited by L Petrillo, BM Bass. New York, Holt, Rinehart, and Winston, 1961.

Hemphill JK, Coons AE: Development of the leader behavior description questionnaire, Leader Behavior: Its Description and Measurement. Edited by R Stogdill, AE Coons. Columbus, Ohio, Ohio State University, Bureau of Business Research, 1957.

Herrold K: Scientific spotlight in leadership, Leadership in Action. Edited by G Lippitt. Washington, National Training Laboratories, National Education Association, 1961.

Hersey P: Blanchard KH: Life cycle theory of leadership. Train Develop J 23(5):26-34, 1969.

Hersey P, Blanchard KH: The management of change: change and the use of power. Train Develop J 26(1):6-10, 1972.

Herzberg F: One more time: how do you motivate employees? Harv Bus Rev 46:53-62, Jan-Feb 1968.

Herzberg F: Work and the Nature of Man. Cleveland, World Publishing Co, 1966.

Higgs Z, Magill K: Nursing leadership needed for our transitional times. J NY State Nurs Assoc 5(3):20-24, 1974.

Hoexter J, McGriff E: Why know how if you don't know what? Nurs Outlook 19(12):794-796, Dec 1971.

Hollander EP: Leaders, Groups, and Influence. New York, Oxford University Press, 1964.

Holloman CR: The nurse enters management. Superv Nurse 2(4):54-67, 1971.

Hopkins T: The Exercise of Influence in Small Groups. Totowa, NJ, Bedminster Press, 1964.

Hospital Research and Educational Trust: Training and Continuing Education, A Handbook for Health Care Institutions. Chicago, Hospital Research and Education Trust, 1970.

House R: Leadership training: some dysfunctional consequences. Admin Sci Q 12:556-571, 1968.

House RJ: A path goal of leader effectiveness. Admin Sci Q 16:321-338, 1971.
Iafolla M: The dilemma of women leaders. Nurs Forum 4(2):54-67, 1965.
Ingalls JD, Arceri JM: A Trainer's Guide to Andragogy. Washington, DC, Department of Health, Education, and Welfare, 1972.
Ingmire A: The effectiveness of a leadership programme in nursing. Int J Nurs Stud 10:3-17, Jan 1973.
Ingmire A, Taylor C: The Effectiveness of a Leadership Program in Nursing. Boulder, Colo, Western Interstate Commission for Higher Education, 1967.
In quest of leadership. Time, July 15, 1974, pp 21-70.
Ivancevich JM, Donnely JH: Leader influence and performance. Personnel Psychol 23:539-549, 1970.
Jacobs TO: Leadership and Exchange in Formal Organizations. Alexandria, Va, Human Resources Research Organization, 1971.
Jacobson WD: Power and Interpersonal Relations. Belmont, Calif, Wadsworth Publishing Company, 1972.
Jacoby J: Creative ability of task-oriented versus person-oriented leaders. J Creative Behav 2:249-253, 1968.
Jaffee CL: Leadership attempting: why and when? Psychol Rep 23:939-946, 1968.
Jay A: Corporation Man. New York, Random House, 1971.
Jelinek R, Munson F, Smith R: SUM (Service Unit Management): An Organizational Approach to Improved Patient Care. Battle Creek, Mich, WK Kellogg Foundation, 1971.
Jennings E: An Anatomy of Leadership: Princes, Heroes, and Supermen. New York, Harper, 1960.
Joel L: The preparation of the nurse in the university setting. J Nurs Ed 11:9-14, January 1972.
Johnson R, Kost F, Rosenzweig J: Systems theory and management, Emerging Concepts of Management. Edited by M Wortman, F Luthans. New York, Macmillan Co., 1969.
Joint Commission for Accreditation of Hospitals: Accreditation Manual. Chicago, Joint Commission for Accreditation of Hospitals, 1970.
Kadushin C: Power, influence, and social circles: a new methodology for studying opinion makers. Am Sociol Rev 33:685-699, 1968.
Kahn RL, Boulding E: Power and Conflict in Organizations. New York, Basic Books, 1964.
Kalisch, BJ: Of half gods and mortals: aesculapian authority. Nurs Outlook 23:22-28, Jan 1975.
Katz R: Skills of an effective administrator. Harv Bus Rev 52:90-102, Sept-Oct 1974.
Kazmier L: Principles of Management. New York, Macmillan Co, 1971.

Keaveny ME: Leadership: What is it? Can the supervisor evaluate it? Superv Nurse 4(1):30-39, 1973.
Kelly DM: Musings on Leadership. Superv Nurse 3:5, Dec 1972.
Kelly RL: Evaluation is more than measurement. Am J Nurs 73:114-116, Jan 1973.
Kelly W: Psychological prediction of leadership in nursing. Nurs Res 23:38-42, Jan-Feb 1974.
Kepner D, Lane WP: Self-confidence in leadership. J Appl Psychol 46: 291-295, 1962.
Knowles M: The Modern Practice of Adult Education. New York, Association Press, 1970.
Koontz E: The Best Kept Secret of the Past 5000 Years: Women are Ready for Leadership in Education. Bloomington, Ind, Phi Delta Kappa, Educational Foundation, 1972.
Koontz H, O'Donnell C: Principles of Management. Fourth edition. New York, McGraw-Hill Publishing Co, 1968.
Korda M: Office power—you are where you sit. New York 8(2):36-44, 1975.
Korda M: Power! How to Get It, How to Use It. New York, Random House, 1975.
Kozma WA, Hirsch I: Commitment, communication enhance programs. Hospitals 46(16):51-54, 1972.
Kramer M, Tegan E, Knaube J: The effect of presets on creative problem solving. Nurs Res 19(4):303-311, July-Aug 1970.
Kron T: Communication in Nursing. Philadelphia, WB Saunders Co, 1967.
Kron T: The Management of Patient Care: Putting Leadership Skills to Work. Philadelphia, WB Saunders Co, 1971.
Lambertsen E: Education for Nursing Leadership. Philadelphia, JB Lippincott Co, 1958.
Lambertsen E: A greater voice for nursing service administrators. Hospitals 46(8):101-108, 1972.
Lansing K: Weaknesses in teacher education. Educ Forum 38:31-39, November 1973.
Leary PA: The Change Agent. Rehab 38(1):30, 1972.
Leavitt H, Pondy, L(eds): Readings in Managerial Psychology. Chicago, University of Chicago Press, 1964.
Lehrer S(ed): Leaders, Teachers and Learners in Academe: Patterns in the Educational Process. New York, Appleton-Century-Crofts, 1970.
Leininger M: The leadership crisis in nursing: a critical problem and challenge. J Nurs Admin 4:28-34, Mar-Apr 1974.
Lemin B: Organizations and their processes. Nurs Times 69(24): 92-96, June 14, 1973.

Lennerlof L: The formal authority of the supervisor. Psychol Res Bull 5(4):2-31, 1965.
Lerner H: Women's liberation. Reflections 9:51-58, 1974.
Levey S, Loomba NP: Health Care Administration—A Managerial Perspective. Philadelphia, JB Lippincott Co, 1973.
Levinson H: Asinine attitudes toward motivation. Harv Bus Rev 51:70-76, Jan-Feb 1973.
Levinson H: The Exceptional Executive. Cambridge, Mass, Harvard University Press, 1968.
Levitt T: The managerial merry-go-round. Harv Bus Rev 52:120-128, July-Aug 1974.
Lewis E: Editorial—Curriculum change: process and product. Nurs Outlook 22:305, May 1974.
Likert R: The Human Organization: Its Management and Value. New York, McGraw-Hill Book Co, 1967.
Lindgren HC: Effective Leadership in Human Relations. New York, Hermitage House, 1954.
Lindquist J, Blackburn R: Middlegrove: the locus of campus power at a state university. AAUP Bull 60:367-68, 1974.
Lippett G(ed): Leadership in Action. Washington, National Training Laboratories, National Education Assoc, 1961.
Lippitt R, Watson J, Westley B: The Dynamics of Planned Change. New York, Harcourt, Brace and World, 1958.
Looking into Nursing Leadership. Leadership in Nursing Monograph, Washington, Leadership Resources Inc, 1966.
Lukens LG: Personality patterns and choice of clinical nursing specialization. Nurs Res, 14:210-221, Summer 1965.
Lynch L: Leadership training in the west. Nurs Outlook 18:38-39, Feb 1970.
Lyons T: Research shows lack of supervisor influence in nursing turnover patterns. Hospitals 44:78-80, Oct 16, 1970.
Mackenzie G, Cory S: Instructional Leadership. New York, Teachers College, Columbia University, Bureau of Publications, 1954.
Mager R, Pipe P: Analyzing Performance Problems. Belmont, Calif, Fearon Publishers, 1970.
Mager R: Goal Analysis. Belmont, Calif, Fearon Publishers, 1972.
Manthey M: Primary care is alive and well in the hospital. Am J Nurs 73:83-87, Jan 1973.
Manthey M, Kramer M: A dialogue on primary nursing. Nurs Forum 9(4):356-379, 1970.
March JG(ed): Handbook of Organizations. Chicago, Rand McNally, 1965.

Maslow A: The Farther Reaches of Human Nature. New York, Viking Press, 1971.
Maslow A: Motivation and Personality. New York, Harper & Row Publishers, 1954.
Mauksch HO: The organization context of nursing practice, The Nursing Profession: Five Sociological Essays. Edited by F. Davis. New York, John Wiley and Sons, 1966.
Mauksch I: Let's listen to the student. Nurs Outlook, 20:103-107, Feb 1975.
McCormack JE: Changing concepts in patient care. Hosp Prog 43:59-62, 1962.
McGannon JB: The academic deanship. Lib Educ 59:277-291, Oct 1973.
McGill University: Nursing Papers, December 1973. Montreal, McGill University School of Nursing, 5(3), 1973.
McGregor C: The Professional Manager. New York, McGraw-Hill Book Co, 1967.
McGregor D: The Human Side of Enterprise. New York, McGraw-Hill Book Co, 1960.
McGregor D: Leadership and Motivation. Cambridge, Mass, MIT Press, 1966.
McGregor D: An uneasy look at performance appraisal. Harv Bus Rev 50(5):133-138, 1972.
McKenney JL, Keen PGW: How managers' minds work. Harv Bus Rev 52:79-90, May-June 1974
McLaughlin F, White E: Small group functioning under six different leadership formats. Nurs Res 22:37-54, Jan-Feb 1973.
McLaughlin FE: Personality changes through alternate group leadership. Nurs Outlook, 20:123-130, Mar-Apr 1971.
McLaughlin FE, Davis ML, Reed JL: Effects of three types of group leadership structure on the self-perceptions of undergraduate nursing students. Nurs Res 21:244-257, May-June 1972.
McMurry RN: Clear communication for chief executives. Harv Bus Rev 43(2):131, 1965.
Megargee EI: Influence of sex roles on the manifestation of leadership. J Appl Psychol 53:377-382, 1969.
Meleis AI, Farrell A: Operation concerning a study of senior nursing students in three nursing programs. Nurs Res 23:461-468, Nov-Dec 1974.
Mercadante L: Leadership development seminars. Nurs Outlook 13:59-61, Sept 1965.
Merton R: The social nature of leadership. Am J Nurs 69:2614-2618, Dec 1969.
Metropolitan Life: Educational attainment and occupations of females. Statist Bull 5:8, Nov 1974.

Miller DI: Education for nursing service administration. Nurs Forum, 7(4):375-385, 1968.
Miller DI: Leaders march to a different drummer. J Nurs Admin 1:3 Jan-Feb 1971.
Miller DI: Standard II: organization is a process. J Nurs Admin 2:19-24, Mar-Apr 1972.
Miner J: Management Theory. New York, Macmillan Co. 1971.
Miner J: The Management Process: Theory, Research, and Practice. New York, Macmillan Co, 1973.
Moloney Sr MA: Leadership behavior of deans in university schools of nursing, unpublished doctoral dissertation, Washington, Catholic University of America, School of Education, 1967.
Moore JC: Social status and social influence: process considerations. Sociometry 32:145-158, 1969.
Moore MA: Philosophy, purpose, and objectives: why do we have them? J Nurs Admin 1(3):9-14, 1971.
Mooth AE, Rivota AE: Developing the Supervisory Skills of the Nurse. New York, Macmillan Co, 1966.
Morphet EL, Johns RL, Reller TL: Educational Organization and Administration. Second edition. Englewood Cliffs, NJ, Prentice Hall, Inc, 1967.
Mott P: Power, authority, and influence, The Structure of Community Power. Edited by M Aiken, P Mott. New York, Random House, 1970.
Murphy AJ: A Study of the leadership process. Am Soc Rev 6:674-687, 1941.
National Center of Health Statistics: Health Resources Statistics 1972-1973. Washington, US Department of Health, Education, and Welfare, Resources Administration, pp 213-229.
National League for Nursing: 1974 NLN Nurse Faculty Census. New York, National League for Nursing, 1975.
National League for Nursing: Some Statistics on Baccalaureate and Higher Degree Programs in Nursing 1973-1974. New York, National League for Nursing, 1975.
National League for Nursing: State Approved School of Nursing RN-1975. New York, National League for Nursing, 1975.
National Student Nurses' Association: NSNA News. New York, Natl Student Nurses' Assoc 5:8, June 1975.
Newcomb TM: The Acquaintance Process. New York, Holt, Rinehart, and Winston, 1961.
New Jersey State Department of Education: The Teaching of Adults. Trenton, NJ, Bureau of Adult Education, New Jersey State Department of Education, undated.
Newman WH, Summer CE: The Process of Management: Concepts, Behavior, Practice. Englewood Cliffs, NJ, Prentice-Hall, 1961.
Nix H: Identification of Leaders and their Involvement in the Planning

Process. Washington, US Department of Health, Education, and Welfare, 1970.
Oaklander H, Fleishman E: Patterns of leadership related to organizational stress in hospital settings. Admin Sci Q 8:520-532, Mar 1964.
O'Brien MJ: Evaluation. Superv Nurs 2(4):24, 31-39, 1971.
Olesen V, Whittaker E: The Silent Dialogue. San Francisco, Jossey-Bass, Inc, 1968.
Owens R: Organizational Behavior in Schools. Englewood Cliffs, NJ, Prentice-Hall, 1970.
Ozimek D: The Future of Nursing Education. New York, National League for Nursing, 1975.
Pattee H(ed): Hierarchy Theory. New York, George Braziller, 1973.
Perrodin C: Supervision of Nursing Service Personnel. New York, Macmillan Co, 1954.
Perrow C: Complex Organizations. Glenview, Ill, Scott, Foresman and Co, 1972.
Perrucci R, Pilisak M: Leaders and ruling elites: the interorganizational bases of community power. Am Sociol Rev 35:1040-1057, 1970.
Peterson GG: The director of nursing should be a nurse. Am J Nurs 73: 1902-1904, Nov 1973.
Petrullo L, Bass BM: Leadership and Interpersonal Behavior. New York, Holt, Rinehart and Winston, 1961.
Pi Lamba Theta: Realizing human potential: focus on women I. Educ Horizons 52:49-103, Winter 1973-1974.
Plott JR: Perception and Change. Ann Arbor, Mich, University of Michigan Press, 1970.
Pryer MW, Distefano MK: Perceptions of leadership behavior, job satisfaction, and internal-external control across three nursing levels. Nurs Res 20:534-541, Nov-Dec 1971.
Raven BH: Social influence and power, Current Studies in Social Psychology. Edited by ID Steiner, M Fishbein. New York, Holt, Rinehart and Winston, 1965.
Richards SA, Cuffe JU: Behavioral correlates of leadership effectiveness in interacting and counteracting groups. J Appl Psychol 56:377-381, Oct 1972.
Rim Y: Leadership attitudes and decisions involving risk. Personnel Psychol 18:423-429, 1965.
Roberts J, Group T: The women's movement and nursing. Nurs Forum 12(3):303-323, 1973.
Rodgers J: Theoretical considerations involved in the process of change. Nurs Forum 12(2):161-174, 1973.
Rogers M: Euphemisms in nursing's future. Image 7(2):3-9, 1975.
Ross MG, Hendry CE: New Understandings of Leadership. New York, Association Press, 1957.

Ross V: An internship for leadership in nursing. Nurs Outlook 14:40-42, Feb 1966.
Rotkovitch R: The director of nursing and the hat of administration. J NY State Nurs Assoc 4:40-43, Nov 1973.
Russell F: The Shadow of Blooming Grove. New York, McGraw-Hill Book Co, 1968.
Sampson RV: The Psychology of Power. New York, Random House, 1968.
Schein E: Process Consultation: Its Role in Organizational Development. Reading, Mass, Addison-Wesley, 1969.
Schwier ME, Gardella FA: Identifying the need for change in nursing service. Nurs Outlook 18:56-62, Apr 1970.
Schwier ME, Gardella FA: Planning, orienting, and preparing for a new kind of nurse leadership. Nurs Outlook 18:42-46, May 1970.
Schlotfeldt R: Knowledge, leaders, and progress. Image 2:2-5, Feb 1968.
Schorr T: Nurse power. Am J Nurs 74:1047, June 1974.
Schurr M: A comparative study of leadership in industry and the nursing profession, part 1, Intern Nurs Rev 16(1):16-29, 1969.
Sears J: The Nature of the Administrative Process. New York, McGraw-Hill Book Co, 1950.
Selvin HC: The Effects of Leadership. New York, Free Press, 1960.
Sexton W: Organization Theories. Columbus, Charles E. Merrill Publishing Co, 1970.
Shanks M, Kennedy D: The Theory and Practice of Nursing Service Administration. New York, McGraw-Hill Book Co, 1965.
Showel M: Interpersonal knowledge and rated leader potential. J Abnorm Soc Psychol 61:87-92, 1960.
Sigma Theta Tau: The Assessment of Leader Behavior. Storrs, Conn, Sigma Theta Tau Headquarters, 1969.
Simms L: Administrative changes and implications for nursing practice in the hospital. Nurs Clin North Am 8:227-234, June 1973.
Simon H: The New Science of Management Decision Making. New York, Harper Brothers, 1960.
Simon H: Administrative Behavior. New York, Macmillan Co, 1959.
Simon H: The organization of complex systems, Hierarchy Theory. Edited by H Pattee. New York, George Braziller, 1973, pp 3-27.
Sirota D, Wolfson AD: Pragmatic approach to people problems. Harv Bus Rev 51:120-128, Jan-Feb 1973.
Smith D: Organizational theory and the hospital. J Nurs Admin 2(3):19-24, 1972.
Smith ML: The clinical specialist: her role in staff development. J Nurs Admin 1:33-34, Jan-Feb 1971.
Smith WP: Precision of control and the use of power in the triad. Hum Relat 21:295-310, 1968.

Somers J: A computerized nursing care system. Hospitals 45:93-100, Apr 1971.
Steinmetz LL: Leadership styles and systems management: more direction, less confusion. Personnel J 47:650-654, 1968.
Stevens B: Analysis of trends in nursing care management. J Nurs Admin 2:12-17, Nov-Dec 1972.
Stevens BJ: The Nurse as Executive. Wakefield, Mass, Contemporary Publishing, Inc, 1975.
Stogdill R: Handbook of Leadership. New York, Free Press, 1974.
Stogdill R: Individual Behavior and Group Achievement. New York, Oxford University Press, 1959.
Stogdill R: The structure of organizational behavior. Multivar Behav Res 2:47-61, 1967.
Stogdill R: Validity of leader behavior descriptions. Personnel Psychol 22:153-158, 1969.
Stogdill R: Personal factors associated with leadership: a survey of the literature. J Psychol 25:35-71, 1948.
Stogdill R, Coons AE: Leader Behavior: Its Description and Measurement. Columbus, Ohio State University, Bureau of Business Research, 1957.
Stogdill R, Goode O, Day R: New Leader behavior description subscales. J Psychol 54:259-269, 1962.
Stogdill R, Scott EL, Jaynes WE: Leadership and Role Expectations. Columbus, Ohio State University, Bureau of Business Research, 1956.
Stogdill R, Shartle CL, Wherry RJ, Jaynes WE: A factorial study of administrative behavior. Personnel Psychol 8:165-180, 1955.
Swansburg RC: Inservice Education. New York, G. P. Putnam's Sons, 1968.
Tannenbaum A: Control in Organization. New York, McGraw-Hill Book Co, 1968.
Tannenbaum R, Schmidt WH: How to choose a leadership pattern. Harv Bus Rev 36:95-101, Mar-Apr 1958.
Tannenbaum R, Schmidt WH: How to choose a leadership pattern. Harv Bus Rev 51(3): 162-164, 167-168, 1973.
Tannenbaum R, Weschler I, Massarik F: Leadership and Organization. New York, McGraw-Hill, 1961.
Tappan F: Toward Understanding Administrators in the Medical Environment. New York, Macmillan Co, 1968.
Tead O: The Art of Administration. New York, McGraw-Hill Book Co, 1951.
The Sexes—women: still number two but trying harder. Time, May 26, 1975, pp 40-41.
Thomas LA: Predicting change in nursing values. J Nurs Admin 1:50-58, May-June 1971.

Thompson L: The nature and need of theory. Educ Forum 39(4): 473-477, 1975.
Thompson V: Modern Organization. New York, Alfred Knopf, 1961.
Titus CH: The Process of Leadership. Dubuque, Iowa, Wm C Brown Co, 1950.
Topf M: A behavioral checklist for estimating the development of communication skills. J Nurs Educ 8(11):29-34, 1969.
Toynbee AJ: Change and Habit. New York, Oxford University Press, 1966.
Udy S: The comparative analysis of organizations. Handbook of Organizations. Edited by J March. Chicago, Rand McNally, 1965, pp 678-709.
U.S. Department of Health, Education and Welfare: The Decanal Role in Baccalaureate and Higher Degree Colleges of Nursing. Washington, DC, US Government Printing Office, 1975.
Vigier F: Change and Apathy. Cambridge, Mass, MIT Press, 1970.
Wallenborn A: Instructional leadership in schools of nursing: what it is and how to prepare for it. Unpublished doctoral dissertation, New York, Teachers College, Columbia University, 1960.
Walsh M, Yura H: Super-Vision, Superv Nurse 2:18-26, Mar 1971.
Weissenberg P, Gruenfeld LW: Relationships among leadership dimensions and cognitive style. J Appl Psychol 40:392-395, 1966.
Weissenberg P, Kavanagh MJ: The independence of initiating structure and consideration: review of the literature. Personnel Psychol 25:119-130, 1972.
Wells LM: The limits of authority: Barnard revisited. Publ Admin Rev 23(3):161-166, 1963.
Wheeler L: Information seeking as a power strategy. J Soc Psychol 62:125-130, 1964.
Wheeler L: Interpersonal Influence. Boston, Allyn and Bacon, 1970.
White B, Barnes B: Power networks in the appraisal process. Harv Bus Rev 49(3):101, 1971.
White H: Some perceived behavior and attitudes of hospital employees under effective and ineffective supervisors. J Nurs Admin 1:49-54, Jan-Feb 1971.
White HC: Perceptions of leadership styles by nurses in supervisory positions. J Nurs Admin 1(2):44-51, 1971.
White M: Importance of selected nursing activities. Nurs Res 21:4-14, Jan-Feb 1972.
Wortman M, Luthans F(eds): Emerging Concepts of Management. New York, Macmillan Co, 1969.
Wrong DH: Some problems in defining social power. Am J Sociol 73:673-681, 1968.
Yale University, School of Nursing Psychiatric Nursing Program: Lead-

ership: problems and possibilities in nursing. Am J Nurs 72:1445-1456, August 1972.

Young L. Room at the top: a place for nurse administrators. J Nurs Admin 2:81-86, Nov-Dec 1972.

Yura H: Faculty perceptions of behavior indicating leadership potential of baccalaureate nursing students, unpublished doctoral dissertation. Washington, The Catholic University of America, School of Education, 1970.

Yura H: Nursing Leadership Behavior. Superv Nurse 2:18-26, Feb 1971.

Yura H, Walsh M: The Nursing Process. New York, Appleton-Century-Crofts, 1973.

Zander A: Motives and Goals in Groups. New York, Academic Press, 1971.

Zollschan GK, Hirsch W: Explorations in Social Change. Boston, Houghton Mifflin, 1964.

Index

Ability, 50
Accountability, 16, 158
Administration, 67–73, 84, 92, 120–22, 136
 theory, 68
Administrative process, 67
Administrator, 7
Advocate, client, 8
Aging, 8
Apprentice, 7
Ashley, J., 57
Assignments, 10
Associate degree programs, 27
Authoritarianism, 24
Authority, 27, 40–47, 48, 49, 51, 58, 61, 64, 74
 definition, 40
 hierarchic 43, 47
 professional, 46, 47

Baccalaureate degree programs, 27, 30, 68, 128–29, 133, 153–57, 198

Baccalaureate degree programs (*cont.*)
 criteria, 135
Barnard, C., 42, 119
Barnes, L., 41, 49
Behavior, 16, 49
Blau, P., 46, 52, 53
Bureaucracy, 24, 44, 45

Cartwright, D., 62
Change, 63, 64, 84, 93, 95, 98, 117
 agent, 60 137
 power, 55
Characteristics, 4, 5, 16, 17, 18, 19, 22, 23, 108, 154–58
Charisma, 3
Coercion, 54, 86
Communication, 59, 86, 88, 91, 95, 98, 108, 115, 166–69, 174
Concept, 11, 47
Continuing education, 128
Control, 50, 53
 hierarchy, 71

233

Coordination, 115
Courage, 3, 5
Criteria
 baccalaureate degree programs, 135
 higher degree programs, 137
Curriculum, improvement, 17

Dalton, G., 41, 42, 48, 49, 63, 64
Deciding, 94, 98, 131
 behavioral counterparts, 139–41
 knowledge delineation, 138–39
 taxonomy, 99
Decision making, 48, 50, 55, 58, 72, 91, 104, 111
 process, 91
Delivery, health care, 16
Democracy, American, 4
Diplomacy, 5
Drucker, P., 2
Duncan, J., 39, 40, 47, 48, 58, 61, 63

Education
 inservice, 128
  situational aspects, 181
 nursing, 6, 29–34, 160–73
 women, 27
Educational programs, 7, 33
 associate degree, 27
 baccalaureate, 27, 30, 68, 128–29, 133, 197
 diploma, 27
 higher degree programs, 29, 133, 137, 197
Ethnic, 5
Etzioni, A., 53

Executives, 2

Facilitating, 94, 98, 106, 107, 131
 behavioral counterparts, 151–52
 knowledge delineation, 149–51
 taxonomy, 101–2
Factors, influential, 15–23
Faculty, 33, 45, 46
Follower, 86, 87, 95, 108, 114, 131

Gardner, J., 134, 196
Gibbs, C., 85, 91
Goal, 7, 15, 59, 84, 86, 92, 95, 108, 114, 116, 131
Graduate nursing education, 129, 157–59
Griffiths, D., 50, 68, 91
Groups, 7, 62, 90, 116–17, 119
Grumbling, 14

Hagen, E., 174–75
Hanlon, J., 198
Hechenberger, N., 160
Hierarchy
 control, 71
 order, 70
 organization, 43, 49, 53, 69, 71, 73, 76
Hospitals, 24, 27

Improvement, curriculum, 17
Influence, 38, 41, 46, 47, 52, 61–65, 85, 88
 definition, 39
 determinants, 62

Index

Influencing, 94, 98, 106, 131
  behavioral counterparts, 147–49
  knowledge delineation, 145–47
  taxonomy, 100–101
Inservice education, 128
  situational aspects, 181
Interpersonal relationships, 62

Jay, A., 119, 121

Kalisch, B., 43
Kaye, E., 172
Kelly, D., 11
Korda, M., 59

Leader, 7, 40, 86, 87, 95, 108
  nurse, 11, 137
Leadership, 2, 118
  characteristic, 4, 5, 16, 17, 18, 19, 22, 23
  definition, 85, 93, 110
  influential factors, 15–23
  nursing, 6, 11, 23, 28, 109
    premises and myths, 102–30
    steps for development, 195–98
  nursing process, 91, 93, 95–98, 113, 117, 118, 120–22, 128, 131
  principles, 92
  research, 82, 197
  shortage, 83
  traitists, 12
  traits, 16–18, 22, 122–24
  types
    autocratic, 9
    democratic, 9, 63
    directive, 9

Learning requisites, 138–52
Leininger, M., 56

Macavity system, 121–22
Management, 72–75, 84, 92, 120–22, 137
Manager, 7
Manipulation, 86
Maslow, A., 14, 177
Massarik, F., 43, 84, 85, 87
Maximizing, 162
McGregor, D., 75, 170
Models, role, 25
Motivation, 14, 114–15, 161, 171, 177
Myths and premises, 102–30

Need satisfaction, 48
Nightingale, F., 25, 84
Nurse practitioners, 10, 175
Nursing, 15
  baccalaureate education, 133, 153–57, 197
  definition, 83, 93, 116
  education, 16, 27, 29–34, 160–73, 197
  goal, 15
  graduate education, 129, 133, 157–59, 197
  process, 94, 127–28
  service, 16, 24–29, 124, 173–92
Nursing leadership, 6, 11, 108
  definition, 93
  myths, 102–30
  premises, 67
  process, 93, 95–98, 113, 117, 120–22, 131
  shortage, 83

Nursing leadership (*cont.*)
  steps for development of, 195–98

Operations, 89
Opinionnaire, 66, 94, 95
  analysis of, 200–214
Order, 70
Organization, 83, 161
  hierarchy, 43, 49, 53, 69, 71, 73

Pattee, H., 69, 71
Performance, definition, 89
Personnel, 28
  auxiliary, 6, 28, 125
Posteriorities, 3
Power, 3, 27, 38, 45, 46, 47–61, 64, 85, 95, 161
  change, 55
  definition, 39, 48, 56
  dimension, 50
  university, 55
Practitioners
  nurse, 10, 175
  professional nursing, 129
  technical nursing, 129
Premises, 102–30
Principles, leadership, 92
Priority, 3
Process, 94
  administrative, 67
  components, 99–102
  decision making, 91
  leadership, 91, 118, 128, 131
  nursing, 94
  nursing leadership, 93, 95–98, 113, 117, 120–22, 127–28, 131
  research, 94

Process (*cont.*)
  supervision, 76
  teaching-learning, 94
Program
  associate degree, 27
  baccalaureate degree, 27, 30, 68, 128–29, 131, 135, 153–57, 197
  continuing education, 128
  educational, 7, 33, 128, 131
  graduate degree, 128, 131, 135, 157–59, 197
  inservice, 128, 181

Qualities, 17

Relating, 94, 98, 105, 131
  behavioral counterparts, 143–45
  knowledge delineation, 141–43
  taxonomy, 99–100
Relationships, 40
  interpersonal, 62
Research, 11, 82, 75, 197
Role, 89, 109, 126
  model, 25

Satisficing, 162
Self-study survey, 135
Sensitivity, 87
Set, 70
Setting, 8
Simon, H., 69
Situation, 85, 87
Social, 19
Statistics, 26–29, 33–34
Steps for development, 195–98

Stogdill, R., 3, 16, 18, 19, 22, 23, 50, 51, 61, 82, 88, 89, 91, 109, 110, 130, 196
Supervision, 53, 72, 75–77, 84, 92, 120–22
Supervisor, 7

Tannenbaum, R., 43, 50, 58, 62, 73, 84, 85, 87
Taxonomy, 99–102
Technical nurse, 129
Territoriality, 59
Theory, 56, 69, 83, 85, 89, 92, 93
   administration, 68
   development, 93
   framework, 30, 39
   nursing, 31–32
   relationship with practice, 31, 32

Theory (*cont.*)
   research, 93
   X and Y, 170
Thompson, V., 42, 197
Traits, 16–18, 22, 122–24

Unit manager, 10

Weschler, I., 43, 84, 85, 87
Wolff, L., 174, 175
Women, 19, 26, 27, 122

Young, L., 26

Zaleznik, A., 41, 49